Contraception Today

A pocketbook for General Practitioners
Fifth edition

John Guillebaud
Emeritus Professor
Family Planning and
Reproductive Health,
University College,
London, UK

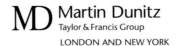

Martin Dunitz
Taylor & Francis Group
LONDON AND NEW YORK

© 1992, 2004 Martin Dunitz, an imprint of the Taylor & Francis Group plc

First published in the United Kingdom in 1992 as *Contraception: Hormonal and Barrier Methods* by
Martin Dunitz, an imprint of the Taylor & Francis Group plc, 11 New Fetter Lane, London EC4P 4EE

Tel.: +44 (0) 20 7583 9855
Fax.: +44 (0) 20 7842 2298
E-mail: info@dunitz.co.uk
Website: http://www.dunitz.co.uk

Fifth edition 2004.

This book represents the personal opinions of John Guillebaud, based wherever possible on published and sometimes unpublished evidence. When (as is not infrequent) no epidemiological or other direct evidence is available, clinical advice herein is always as practical and realistic as possible and based, pending more data, on the author's judgement of other sources. These may include the opinions of Expert Committees and any existing Guidelines. In some instances the advice appearing in this book may even so differ appreciably from the latter, for reasons usually given in the text and (since medical knowledge and practice are continually evolving) relates to the date of publication. Healthcare professionals must understand that they take ultimate responsibility for their patient and ensure that any clinical advice they use from this book is applicable to the specific circumstances that they encounter.

A CIP record for this book is available from the British Library.

ISBN 1 84184 386 5

Distributed in the USA by
Fulfilment Center
Taylor & Francis
10650 Toebben Drive
Independence, KY 41051, USA
Toll Free Tel.: +1 800 634 7064
E-mail: taylorandfrancis@thomsonlearning.com

Distributed in Canada by
Taylor & Francis
74 Rolark Drive
Scarborough, Ontario M1R 4G2, Canada
Toll Free Tel.: +1 877 226 2237
E-mail: tal_fran@istar.ca

Distributed in the rest of the world by
Thomson Publishing Services
Cheriton House
North Way
Andover, Hampshire SP10 5BE, UK
Tel.: +44 (0)1264 332424
E-mail: salesorder.tandf@thomsonpublishingservices.co.uk

Composition by Wearset Ltd, Boldon, Tyne and Wear

Printed and bound in Italy by Printer Trento

Statement of competing interests
The author has received payments for research projects, lectures, *ad hoc* consultancy work and related expenses from the manufacturers of contraceptive products.

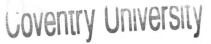

Contents

Preface

We have not inherited the earth from our grandparents, we have borrowed it from our grandchildren.

Attributed to the ancient Chinese

Family planning could bring more benefits to more people at less cost than any other single technology now available to the human race.

UNICEF, 1992

Born and reared in Burundi and Rwanda, countries whose agonies are in significant measure related to excessive population growth, I maintain that:

Human **needs** along with those of all other species with which we share the Natural World will never be sustainably met on a finite planet without more concerned, non-coercive, action on human **numbers**.

No woman on earth who at time present wishes to exercise her human right to have control of her fertility should be denied the means to do so, by any agency – whether her partner, her society, or the inadequacy or cost of the supplies and services available to her.

In their life-time, every new birth in the UK is likely, through the inevitable effluence of his or her affluence as a consumer, to harm the environment as much as 30–200 births in Burundi or Bangladesh will ever have the opportunity to do. We all have a part to play in ensuring that our grandchildren receive back their "loan" in a halfway decent and long-term sustainable state (see www.ecotimecapsule.com). As a small but relevant contribution to that endeavour, I welcome this opportunity to bring a new edition of this pocketbook on contraception to general practioners and nurses in Primary Care.

I write, moreover, as one who is proud to have worked in general practice, as a locum in places as diverse as Barnsley, Cambridge, Luton and South London, and hence able to appreciate some of the satisfactions and the constraints of that role.

John Guillebaud.

September 2003

John Guillebaud is Emeritus Professor of Family Planning and Reproductive Health at University College London, Honorary Consultant in Family Planning for the Oxford Community Primary Care Trust and Co-Chair of the Optimum Population Trust.

Until 2002 he was also Medical Director of the Margaret Pyke Centre in London, and continues as a Trustee of the Margaret Pyke Memorial Trust.

Acknowledgements

I wish to thank numerous friends and colleagues in the UK and abroad working in relevant specialist and general practice – too many to mention all by name. Toni Belfield, Head of Information at the UK FPA, Dr Anne MacGregor, MPC's Medical Adviser, and Alison Campbell, Ian Mellor and Robert Peden of the Martin Dunitz Imprint who have guided this work now through 5 editions, do however deserve special mention. I acknowledge much help over the years from senior medical and nursing staff at the Margaret Pyke Centre (MPC) and am also grateful to some of our clients for the insights they have given me.

Introduction

General practitioners (GPs) are often best placed to offer good contraceptive advice because they already know the patient's health and family circumstances. Some practices are excellent; others provide little beyond oral contraception and devote insufficient time and skill to counselling. The 2002 Sexual Health Strategy established that primary care should always supply at least Level 1 basic contraceptive services, and be fully organized to refer as appropriate to services at Level 2 [including the fitting of implants and intrauterine devices (IUDs) or the intrauterine system (IUS)] or Level 3 (male and female sterilization, legal abortion). Women with more complex contraceptive or sexual problems may be asked to re-attend after surgery. Much can, indeed should, be delegated to a practice nurse fully trained in family planning, usually with a gain rather than a loss in standards. Practice is changing fast, with more use of patient group directions and more trained nurse prescribers and practitioners, some of whom insert intrauterine and subdermal contraceptives. Aside from those, who are still relatively few, a good mainstream practice nurse may appropriately perform the following delegated functions:

- Taking sexual and medical history, discussion of choices
- Cap fitting, checking, teaching
- Pill teaching
- Pill issuing/reissuing and emergency pill issuing – given fully agreed and audited patient group directions
- Pill monitoring [including migraine assessment and blood pressure (BP)]
- Contraceptive injections [Depo Provera (DMPA)™ (Pharmacia & Upjohn)]
- IUD and IUS checking, including for cervical excitation tenderness
- Cervical smear taking

Formal training is also desirable for doctors* and should include both theoretical and 'apprenticeship' training, as well as discussion of the often complex psychosexual and emotional factors involved in the use of contraception. All clinicians should be sensitive to hidden signals in this area.

Doctors should back their counselling with good literature. Although some manufacturers have improved their package labelling, the latest UK Family Planning Association (FPA) leaflets are better – user-friendly, yet accurate and comprehensive. The one called *Your Guide to Contraception* tabulates all the important methods, both reversible and permanent, and is ideal for reading in the waiting room before counselling. The leaflets on individual methods, especially *Your Guide to the Combined Pill*, should be given with advice to 'read, and keep long term for further reference'. The month and date of publication should be recorded in the patient's notes. Follow-up patients may need a replacement. Together with accurate contemporary records, these leaflets – being fully revised in the light of World Health Organization

* In the UK, the Faculty of Family Planning and Reproductive Health Care (in this book termed 'the Faculty of FP') offers, through agencies such as the Margaret Pyke Centre (MPC), educational courses for doctors leading to their Diploma (DFFP) and Membership (MFFP), as well as Letters of Competence in Intrauterine Techniques, Subdermal Implants and Instructing. In 2002, nurses and associate practitioners working in reproductive health became eligible to become Associates of the Faculty. The Institute of Psychosexual Medicine offers relevant seminar training.

(WHO) advice in the autumn of 2003 – provide strong medicolegal back-up for practitioners who may be asked to justify their actions in the event of litigation. They are an essential supplement to – but by no means a replacement for – time spent with the health care practitioner.

Choice of method

Most women who seek contraception are healthy and young, and present fewer problems than the over-35s, teenagers and those with intercurrent disease. There is an increasing tendency for sterilization procedures to be demanded at too early an age. This is partly because the Pill is too often seen as synonymous with contraception, and we as providers have not been informing women about the many new or improved reversible alternatives to

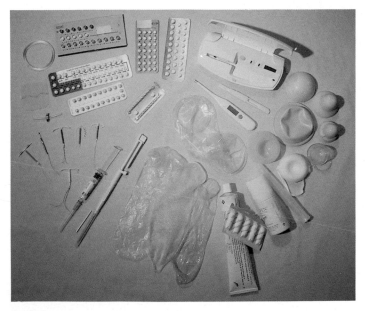

Figure 1
The choice of methods in the UK. (Reproduced with kind permission of Dr Anne MacGregor.)

the Pill and condom, about which there is still much ignorance and mythology. See Figure 1. I refer particularly to the levonorgestrel IUS (LNG IUS), the T-Safe Cu 380A, the GyneFix, injectables and the latest implants.

The very young

I am opposed to sex education. What we should say, and promote, is sex and relationships education (SRE). When seeking advice on sex, relationships, contraception, pregnancy and parenthood, young people are entitled to accessible, confidential, non-judgemental and unbiased support and guidance – recognizing the diversity of their cultural and faith traditions. We should listen to their views and respect their opinions and choices. Valid choices include not having as well as having (safer and contracepted) sex.

However, as they may often 'get away with it' in one or more cycles, all too often the young do not seek advice until they have already conceived. Easier access to emergency contraception is an obvious priority. But education must promote (as in the Netherlands) the societal norm that sex may be a feature of a good relationship only when and if adequate contraception exists. In this age group we still await as first-line more 'forgettable' methods in which (in contrast to the Pill) non-pregnancy is the default state. Injectables and implants are usually preferable to copper IUDs because they provide some protection against pelvic infection, although IUDs are only relatively contraindicated (the GyneFix or LNG IUS may also be appropriate).

In spite of not having the ideal default state, for many young women the most suitable initial method currently remains a modern, low-oestrogen, combined oral contraceptive (COC) – or the new progestogen-only pill (POP) Cerazette™ – backed by good counselling.

With patients under 16 years of age it remains reasonable

– so long as it is done opportunely, non-judgementally and in a non-patronizing way – to present the emotional, physical and legal advantages of delaying intercourse (and then of mutually faithful relationships). But if that is 'best', when it is rejected it must not become the enemy of 'good', a category that surely includes contraception (with age-appropriate SRE which ideally begins in the home). Involvement of at least one parent is vastly preferable to that of neither, yet it can be good practice to prescribe the Pill without it (see Box below). *At all times the young woman must be assured of confidentiality.*

There is a useful mnemonic for the UK Memorandum of Guidance [DHSS HC(FP)86] regarding under 16s, issued after the Gillick case.

Mnemonic: UnProtected SSexual InterCourse. The health care practitioner:	

U	Must ensure the young person **UNDERSTANDS** the potential risks and benefits of the treatment/advice given
P	Is legally obliged to discuss the value of **PARENTAL** support, yet the client must know that confidentiality is respected whether or not this is given
S	Should assess whether the client is likely to have **SEXUAL** intercourse without contraception
S	Should assess whether the young person's physical/mental health may **SUFFER** if not given contraceptive advice or supplies
I	Must consider if it is in the client's best **INTERESTS** to give contraception without parental consent
C	Must respect the duty of **CONFIDENTIALITY** that should be given to a person under 16, and which is as great as that owed to any other person

Note: Available free from the RCOG or the Royal College of Nursing (RCN) since 2002 is an invaluable laminated leaflet called Getting it Right for Teenagers in Your Practice.

Sexually transmitted infections

Always take a quick but matter-of-fact sexual history: an excellent screening question is: 'When did you last have sex with someone different?' Advise the sexually active of all ages about minimizing their risk of sexually transmitted infections (STIs), including the human immunodeficiency virus (HIV). Besides 'selling' monogamy on medical grounds *it is essential to promote the condom as an addition to the selected contraceptive whenever infection risk exists – the so-called Double-Dutch approach.*

Relative effectiveness of available methods

Good results depend on a couple-based, individualized approach – contraception is very much about choosing 'horses for courses'. Iatrogenic pregnancies can frequently be caused by avoidable omissions and errors on the part of service providers. Table 1 outlines the comparative efficacy of most current methods.

Unwanted effects of contraceptives: contraindications

These are obviously important issues, but risks must be impartially evaluated (a failing of the mass media) and then rationally applied as contraindications without introducing unjustified medical barriers to contraceptive use.

An important general principle is *summation*, discussed on p. 41. Also helpful is the WHO system for classifying contraindications, which is applied in this book (to the best of my judgement). It is an evidence-based system, where evidence exists, but also tries to give the best interim guidance when we have to make a decision (in consultation with the woman/couple), in the frustrating absence of good evidence. This scheme (which I had a hand in devising at a WHO meeting in Atlanta in 1994) is more fully

Table 1
First-year user-failure rates per 100 women for different methods of contraception.

Method of contraception	Range in the world literature*	Oxford/FPA study (Lancet report in 1982; all women married and aged above 25)	
		Age 25–34 (≤2 years' use)	Age 35+ (≤2 years' use)
Sterilization			
Male (after azoospermia)	0–0.05	0.08	0.08
Female	0–0.5	0.45	0.08
Subcutaneous implant			
Implanon	0–0.07		
Injectable (DMPA)	0–1	–	–
Combined pills			
50 µg oestrogen	0.1–3	0.25	0.17
<50 µg oestrogen	0.2–3	0.38	0.23
EVRA contraceptive patch	0.6–0.9		
Cerazette (POP)	0.2–0.9		
Progestogen-only pill	0.3–4	2.5	0.5
Intrauterine contraception			
Levonorgestrel intrauterine system (LNG IUS)	0–0.6		
IUDs			
T-Safe Cu 380A	0.3–0.8		
GyneFix	0.1–1.2		
Other > 300 mm copper IUDs, unbanded (e.g. Nova T380, Multiload 375, Flexi T300)	0.2–1.5		
Diaphragm	4–20	5.5	2.8
(Male) condom	2–15	6.0	2.9
Female condom	5–15		
Coitus interruptus	6–17	–	–
Spermicides alone	4–25	–	–
Fertility awareness	2–25	–	–
'Persona'	6–?	–	–
No method, young women	80–90	–	–
No method at age 40	40–50	–	–
No method at age 45	10–20	–	–
No method at age 50 (if still having menses)	0–5	–	–

*Excludes atypical studies and all extended use studies. For sterilization, the rates in second column are estimated **lifetime failure rates**. Re Filshie clip, visit www.rcog.org.uk.

Note: 1. First figure of range in second column gives a rough measure of 'perfect use' (but is not the same).

         2. Influence of age, all the rates in the fourth column being lower than those in the third column. Lower rates still may be expected above the age of 45.

         3. Much better results also obtainable in other states of relative infertility, e.g. lactation.

         4. Oxford/FPA users were established users as recruitment, greatly improving results especially for barrier methods.

         5. *Caution:* The Implanon™, EVRA™ and Cerazette results are different. They come from pre-marketing studies, giving an estimate of the Pearl "method-failure" rate and the upper bound of the 95% confidence interval.

described in two WHO documents on medical eligibility criteria [WHO (2000) *Medical Eligibility Criteria for Contraceptive Use* (WHO/RHR/00.02) (2nd edn, 2001) and WHO (2002) *Selected Practice Recommendations for Contraceptive Use* (ISBN: 92 4 154566 6)]. There are now four categories of contraindication, considered in the Box below.

WHO Classification of contraindications*
1. A condition for which there is no restriction for the use of the contraceptive method
  'A' is for **Always Usable**
2. A condition where the advantages of the method generally outweigh the theoretical or proven risks
  'B' is for **Broadly Usable**
3. A condition where the theoretical or proven risks usually outweigh the advantages, so an alternative method is usually preferred. Yet, respecting the patient/client's autonomy, if she accepts the risks and rejects or should not use relevant alternatives, given the risks of pregnancy the method can be used with caution/sometimes with additional monitoring
  'C' is for **'Caution/Counselling'**, if used at all
4. A condition which represents an unacceptable health risk
  'D' is for **'DO NOT USE'**, at all

---

* My A–D additions are *aide-mémoires*. WHO 1–4 numbering is used in this book to avoid confusion.

The most useful new feature of the classification is the separation into two categories of 'Relative' contraindication (WHO 2 and 3).

Clinical judgement is required, always in consultation with the contraceptive user, especially: (1) In all WHO 3 conditions; or (2) If more than one condition applies. As a working rule, two WHO 2 conditions move the situation to WHO 3; and if any WHO 3 condition applies the addition of either a 2 or a 3 condition normally means WHO 4, i.e. 'Do not use'.

Combined hormonal contraception

COMBINED ORAL CONTRACEPTIVES
Mechanism of action

Aside from secondary contraceptive effects on the cervical mucus and to impede implantation, combined oral contraceptives (COCs) primarily prevent ovulation. They therefore remove the normal menstrual cyle and replace it with a cycle which is user-produced and based only on the end organ, i.e. the endometrium. So the withdrawal bleeding has minimal medical significance, can be deliberately postponed or made infrequent (e.g. tricycling, see p. 58), and if it fails to occur, once pregnancy is excluded, poses no problem. The pill-free time is the contraception-deficient time, which has great relevance to maintenance of the COC's efficacy (see below).

Benefits versus risks

COCs can provide virtually 100% protection from unwanted pregnancy. They can be taken at a time unconnected with intercourse and provide enormous reassurance by the regular, short, light and usually painless withdrawal bleeding at the end of each pack. Most of the discussion here concerns possible risks* but the positive aspects should not be forgotten.

* Data derived mainly from the prospective Royal College of General Practitioners (RCGP), Oxford/FPA and US Nurses Studies, supplemented by numerous case–control studies conducted by WHO and other bodies.

Contraceptive benefits of COCs.
- Effectiveness
- Convenience, not intercourse related, 'forgettability'
- Reversibility

Non-contraceptive benefits of COCs.
- Reduction of most menstrual cycle disorders: less heavy bleeding, therefore less anaemia, and less dysmenorrhoea; regular bleeding, the timing of which can be controlled (no Pill-taker need have 'periods' at weekends; upon request, she may tricycle and so bleed only a few times a year, see p. 58): fewer symptoms of premenstrual tension overall; no ovulation pain
- Fewer functional ovarian cysts because abnormal ovulation is prevented
- Fewer extrauterine pregnancies because normal ovulation is inhibited
- Reduction in pelvic inflammatory disease (PID)
- Reduction in benign breast disease
- Fewer symptomatic fibroids
- Probable reduction in thyroid disease (both overactive and underactive syndromes)
- Probable reduction in risk of rheumatoid arthritis
- Fewer sebaceous disorders (with oestrogen-dominant COCs)
- Possibly fewer duodenal ulcers (not well established and perhaps due to avoidance of COCs by anxious women)
- Reduction in *Trichomonas vaginalis* infections
- Possible lower incidence of toxic shock syndrome
- Reduced risk of cancers of ovary and endometrium (see text), and possibly also colorectal cancer
- No toxicity in overdose
- Obvious beneficial social effects

Even as we turn to unwanted effects, it is reassuring that, according to the RCGP report in 1999, COCs have their main (small) effect on every associated cause of mortality during current use and for some (variable) time thereafter. The excess thrombotic risk has probably vanished by 4 weeks and by 10 years after use ceases, mortality in past-users is indistinguishable from that in never-users.

Tumours

Breast cancer

This has a high incidence and therefore it must inevitably be expected to develop in women whether or not they use COCs. As recognized risk factors for breast cancer include early menarche and late age of first birth, use of COCs by young women was bound to receive scientific scrutiny. However, increasing age is the most important risk factor (Figure 2), so if there is a real causative link with use of the Pill, use by older women will obviously lead to more attributable cases.

The 1996 publication by the Collaborative Group on Hormonal Factors in Breast Cancer (CGHFBC) proposed a model which is the one now most widely accepted. The group reanalysed original data from over 53 000 women with breast cancer and over 100 000 controls from 54 studies in 25 countries. This was 90% of the worldwide epidemiological data to that date.

The CGHFBC's model shows disappearance of the risk in ex-users, but now 'recency of use' of the COC is the most

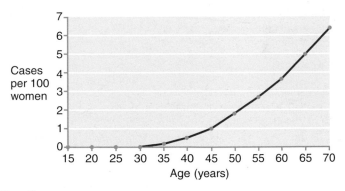

Figure 2
Background risk: cumulative number of breast cancers per 100 women, by age. (Reproduced from statement by Faculty of Family Planning, June 1996.)

important factor, with the odds ratio unaffected by age of initiation or discontinuation, use before or after first full-term pregnancy, or duration of use. The main findings are summarized in Table 2.

Table 2
The increased risk of developing breast cancer while taking the pill and in the 10 years after stopping (CGHFBC Lancet 1996; 347: 1713–27).

User status	Increased risk
Current user	24%
1–4 years after stopping	16%
5–9 years after stopping	7%
10 plus years an ex-user	No significant excess

COC users can be reassured that:

- While the small increase in breast cancer risk for women on the pill noted in previous studies is confirmed, the odds ratio of 1.24 signifies an increase of 24% only while women are taking the COC and for a few years thereafter, diminishing to zero after 10 years
- As Figure 2 shows, breast cancer is fortunately very rare in women under-35 and since most Pill usage is also completed by that age, the attributable increased risk from 24% is very small
- Beyond 10 years after stopping the Pill there is no detectable increase in breast cancer risk. This is now confirmed in a 2002 US study by Marchbanks to apply even in those exposed young or before a first full-term pregnancy. There is no time bomb of cancer risk delayed many years after ceasing Pill use
- The cancers diagnosed in women who use or have ever used COCs are clinically less advanced than in those who have never used the Pill and are less likely to have spread beyond the breast
- The CGHFBC reanalysis showed that these risks are not associated with duration of use or the dose or type of hormone in the COC, and that there is no synergism with other risk factors for breast cancer (e.g. family history – see p. 15)
- The apparent risks for users of POP and injectables are similar to those using COC, but failed to reach statistical significance

The collaborative group conceded that its findings in ever-takers of the Pill, of less advanced cases being identified but more of them at each given age, suggested surveillance bias; and the latter might even explain all or part of the findings in current users as well. However, the consensus interpretation which I personally accept for the present is that the pill is a weak cofactor for breast cancer in young current and recent users, but that for some reason the resulting tumours are less aggressive.

Clinical implications

The Faculty of FP in the UK states that users of the Pill should be informed of/counselled about the above data, but reiterates the advice of the UK Committee on the Safety of Medicines that otherwise prescribing practice should not change.

The breast cancer issue is part of routine pill counselling, the discussion being initiated opportunely – often not at the first visit unless raised by the woman – along with encouragement to report promptly any unusual changes in the breasts at any time in the future ('breast awareness'). The balancing protective effects against malignancy of the ovary and endometrium (see below) should also be mentioned. *The known contraceptive and non-contraceptive benefits of COCs may seem so great to many (but not to all) as to compensate for almost any likely lifetime excess risk of breast cancer.*

Figure 3 helps to summarize the situation. Imagine a concert hall (Hall 1) filled with 1000 Pill-users, all *now aged 45* but all having used a COC for varying durations of time, then *having stopped by the age of 35* (a common situation). The (cumulative) number of cases of breast cancer would be 11. However, in a similar auditorium (Hall 2 – not illustrated) filled with never-takers of the Pill, also all aged 45, there would be 10 cases, i.e. there is only one

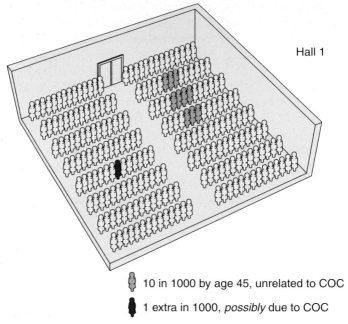

Hall 1

👤 10 in 1000 by age 45, unrelated to COC

👤 1 extra in 1000, *possibly* due to COC

Figure 3
Cumulative incidence of breast cancer during and after use of COC until age 35.

Pill-attributable case, allowing for Pill use of any duration to year of age 35 plus 10 years' post-use. Moreover:

- If the Pill is acting as a cofactor, not initiator, for breast cancer then it is possible that the one excess case is a woman who would have developed the disease without the Pill anyway, but at a later age
- The remaining 989 ex-Pill-users will from this time on have only the same risk of breast cancer as other women now aged 45, i.e. there is no ongoing added risk because it is over 10 years since they last took the Pill. This is a very important finding given that the overall risk of breast cancer rises significantly with age
- The cancers diagnosed among Pill-users (current and in the next 10 years), also tend to be less advanced than those in Hall 2

What about Pill use by the older woman, or in *WHO 2 risk groups for breast cancer?* Specifically: (1) women with a family history of a young (under 40 years of age), first-degree relative with breast cancer and (2) women with benign breast disease (BBD) *without* pre-malignant epithelial atypia on histology. (If present, the latter is WHO 4 i.e. 'Do not use'.)

Older women are now permitted to use COC to about the age of 51 – the mean age of the menopause – if they so choose, provided they are healthy, migraine-free, non-smokers. The cumulative risk of breast cancer in young women is very small, being 2 in 1000 in women up to the age of 35, but it increases with age thereafter, to 10 in 1000 at the age of 45 and 80 in 1000 by the age of 75 (see Figure 2). *If the background risk for the individual is larger, whether because of increased age, uncomplicated BBD or a family history*, the percentage increment (24%) during current use does not increase. However, *applied to a bigger background risk it will obviously mean more attributable cases* (e.g. an extra 3 in a 1000 with Pill-use to the age of 45) than in younger women without any risk factors for breast cancer. Therefore, these are **relative contraindications** (usually WHO 2), which require careful explanation. If the woman chooses COC – as she is en-titled to do, given its contraceptive advantages and pro-tection against cancer of the ovary and endometrium (see below) – it should be a low-dose formulation, with specific counselling, extra surveillance and periodic reassess-ment.

If carcinoma of the breast develops, the prognosis is good in Pill-users; however, COCs should be stopped and an alternative effective method such as an IUD arranged. Low-dose progestogen-only methods are an option (WHO 3), after consultation with the woman's oncologist, pro-vided the woman is in remission (for five years according to the WHO itself).

Cervical cancer

Studies of cervical cancer are always complicated by a lack of accurate information on sexual activity of women and especially their partners. Human papilloma virus (HPV) types 16 and 18 are important candidates as the principal carcinogen, which is clearly transmitted sexually. A 2003 review of the studies – including those which identified and controlled for the presence of HPV – leads to the conclusion that the COC may act as a cofactor, speeding transition through all stages of cervical intraepithelial neoplasia (CIN). In this respect it is similar to, but certainly weaker than, cigarette smoking.

Clinical implications.
- Prescribers must of course ensure that Pill-users are adequately screened following agreed guidelines. Even if they also smoke, a 3-yearly smear frequency is still believed to suffice to identify and treat appropriately the vast majority (not all) in pre-invasive stages, before actual cancer develops
- It is acceptable practice (WHO 2) to continue COC use during the careful monitoring of any abnormality, or after definitive treatment of CIN.

Liver tumours

COC use increases the relative risk of **benign adenoma** or **hamartoma**, which can cause pain or a haemoperitoneum. However, the background incidence is so small (1–3 per 1 million women per year) that the COC-attributable risk is minimal. Most reported cases have been in long-term users of relatively high-dose pills.

Three case-control studies also support the view that the rare **primary hepatocellular carcinoma** is less rare in COC users than it is in controls. However, although it is usually fatal within one year it is reasuring that the death-rate from this cancer has not changed detectably in the US or Sweden where the COC has been widely used since the 1960s. Moreover there is no evidence of synergism with either cirrhosis or hepatitis B liver infection.

Choriocarcinoma

In the presence of active trophoblastic disease, UK studies have shown that chemotherapy for choriocarcinoma is more often required among women given COCs. This has not been shown in studies from the US, probably because chemotherapy there is given to almost all cases of trophoblastic disease, thereby obliterating any hormonal effect.

Clinical implications

- When any form of trophoblastic disease has been diagnosed, although WHO classifies this as WHO 1, in the UK it is still recommended by the regional centres that monitor all cases that all sex steroids should be avoided (WHO 4) while human chorionic gonadotrophin (hCG) levels are raised. This advice includes the progestogen-only methods, but emergency contraception (EC) is permitted (WHO 3)
- What contraception should be used until hCG is undetectable? Fortunately, while hCG levels are above 5000 IU/l ovulation is very improbable so barrier methods should be effective (IUDs are also usable, usually after preliminary imaging to exclude invasive damage to the uterine wall from cancer)
- After the all-clear has been given by the regional centre, any hormonal method is usable (WHO 1)

Carcinomas of the ovary and of the endometrium

The good news is that both are definitely less frequent in COC-users. Numerous studies have shown that the incidence of both is roughly halved among all users, and reduced to one third in long-term users; a protective effect can be detected in ex-users for up to 10–15 years. Suppression of ovulation and of normal menstruation in COC-users probably explains these findings.

Other cancers

Other links (e.g. possible promotion of the endometrioid type of intracervical cancer but protection against colorectal cancer) have been mooted.

Benefits and risks – a summary for cancer

In counselling, a balance exists (Figure 4). Since the 4th edition of this book in 2000, a question mark has been removed from cancer of the cervix but remains before breast cancer (since the apparent co-factor effect in younger women still could be due to surveillance bias). Computer modelling suggests that populations using COCs may develop different benign or malignant neoplasms from control populations, but there is a distinct possibility (without proof) that the overall risk of death from neoplasia is reduced.

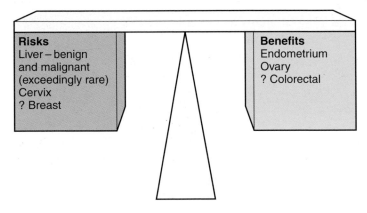

Risks
Liver – benign
and malignant
(exceedingly rare)
Cervix
? Breast

Benefits
Endometrium
Ovary
? Colorectal

Figure 4
Cancer and COCs: a balance.

Circulatory disease and choice of COC

The objective of prescribing is efficacy with maximum safety, and with the Pill this primarily means safety in relation to arterial and venous circulatory disease. This safety depends on choosing appropriate users as much as the appropriate Pill. The following is a useful framework for this process:

1. What are the benefits versus the risks? (Discussed above, and pp. 27–9)
2. Who should never take the Pill? (**absolute contraindications**; pp. 37–9)
3. Who usually should not take the Pill? Maybe, but then with special advice, alertness to synergism and monitoring (**relative contraindications and interacting diseases**; pp. 30–1, 34–5, 39ff)
4. Which are the safer pills?
5. What are the guidelines for prescribing (Tables 5 & 6 and pp. 29–37)?
6. Which is the second choice of pill?
7. What is necessary for monitoring during follow-up?
   - BP
   - headaches, especially migraines
   - management of important new risk factors or diseases
   - management of minor side effects
   - implications of the pill-free week

Risk factors for circulatory disease are of greatest relevance, and the research available since 1995 means we should now consider *separately* for each woman the risk factors for venous and arterial thrombosis (pp. 30–1, 34–5). Questions (2) and (3) identify the 'dangerous' women, or rather the 'most unsafe' and the 'less unsafe' women respectively, for the Pill. The answers are pivotal in answering the next questions in this sequence:

4. Which are the 'safer' pills?
5. What are the guidelines for prescribing (pp. 29–37)?

All modern low-dose COCs contain ethinylestradiol (EE) combined with a variety of progestogens (Figure 5 and Table 3). Note that there are six main 'ladders' of progestogens, since *in vivo* norethisterone acetate (NETA) is converted with great efficiency to norethisterone (NET). These progestogens are usefully classified into two groups. The first is often, but unhelpfully, referred to as second generation (LNG and NET with its prodrugs). The other group is the remainder, including those with desogestrel (DSG) and gestodene (GSD) – formerly termed third generation – but also drospirenone (DSP) and (not displayed in Figure 5) cyproterone acetate (CPA). Norgestimate (NGM) as in Cilest™ (Janssen-Cilag), with 35 μg of EE, is, in my view, *effectively* also in this group (see p. 37) of formulations, which are all more **oestrogen-dominant** than LNG- or NET-containing products.

The intention when first prescribing is, taking account of any risk factors or interacting diseases, to minimize adverse effects of both components of the Pill: by giving the lowest acceptable dose of oestrogen and allowing for differences in known biological effects of the progestogens. In simple terms, smaller pills give smaller side effects.

---

6. Which is the second choice of pill?

Details follow, but in general this means:

- For *bleeding side effects,* using endometrial bleeding as, to a limited degree, a biological assay of the contraceptive steroids (see pp. 47–9)
- For the common *non-bleeding minor side effects,* making (mostly on empirical grounds) changes to the formulation used (pp. 49–50)

Venous thromboembolism (VTE)

The dust has at last settled on the media hype and 'Pill scare' which followed a letter from the UK Committee on the Safety of Medicines (CSM) on 18 October 1995, based on congruent but at the time unpublished studies. At the time many of us wished that the story had been officially presented as a *reduction* of risk of VTE if women used LNG or NET pills. I see this as not only a matter of presentation, explaining to the public and the media that 'the bottle is half full, rather than half empty'. It is also

Table 3 *Formulations of currently marketed combined oral contraceptives (COCs).*

Pill type	Preparation	Oestrogen (µg)	Progestogen (µg)	
Monophasic				
Ethinylestradiol/ norethisterone type	Loestrin 20	20	1000	Norethisterone acetate*
	Loestrin 30	30	1500	Norethisterone acetate*
	Brevinor	35	500	Norethisterone
	Ovysmen	35	500	Norethisterone
	Norimin	35	1000	Norethisterone
Ethinylestradiol/ levonorgestrel	Microgynon 30 (also ED)	30	150	
	Ovranette	30	150	
	Eugynon 30	30	250	
Ethinylestradiol/ desogestrel	Mercilon	20	150	
	Marvelon	30	150	
Ethinylestradiol/ gestodene	Femodette	20	75	
Ethinylestradiol/ gestodene	Femodene (also ED)	30	75	
	Minulet	30	75	
Ethinylestradiol/ norgestimate	Cilest	35	250	
Ethinylestradiol drospirenone	Yasmin	30	3000	
Mestranol/ norethisterone	Norinyl-1	50	1000	
Bi/triphasic				
Ethinylestradiol/ norethisterone	BiNovum	35	500 } 833†	(7 tabs)
		35	1000	(14 tabs)
	Synphase	35	500	(7 tabs)
		35	1000 } 714	(9 tabs)
		35	500	(5 tabs)
	TriNovum	35	500	(7 tabs)
		35	750 } 750	(7 tabs)
		35	1000	(7 tabs)
Ethinylestradiol/ levonorgestrel	Logynon (also ED)	30 } 32†	50	(6 tabs)
		40	75 } 92	(5 tabs)
		30	125	(10 tabs)
	Trinordiol	30 } 32	50	(6 tabs)
		40	75 } 92	(5 tabs)
		30	125	(10 tabs)
Ethinylestradiol/ gestodene	Tri-Minulet	30 } 32	50	(6 tabs)
		40	70 } 79	(5 tabs)
		30	100	(10 tabs)
	Triadene	30 } 32	50	(6 tabs)
		40	70 } 79	(5 tabs)
		30	100	(10 tabs)
Ethinylestradiol/ cyproterone acetate	Dianette‡	35	2000	

*Converted to norethisterone as the active metabolite.
†Equivalent daily doses for comparison with monophasic brands.
‡Marketed primarily as acne therapy (see text) – and not intended to be used as a routine pill.
Other names worldwide are on website www.ippf.org.uk

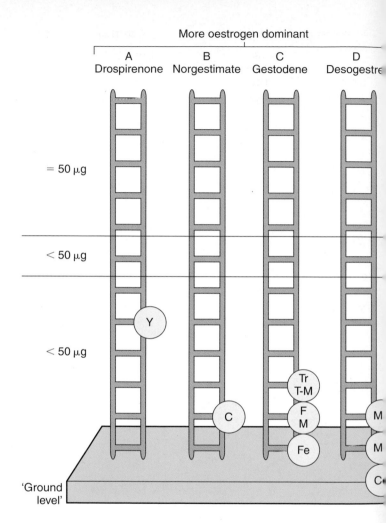

Figure 5
COC formulations available in the UK.
Note: ED or every day means placebos are given on pill-free days.

Ladder A
Y = Yasmin
Ladder B
C = Cilest
Ladder C
Tr = Triadene
T-M = Tri-Minulet

F = Femodene (also ED)
M = Minulet
Fe = Femodette
Ladder D
Ma = Marvelon
Me = Mercilon
Ce = Cerazette

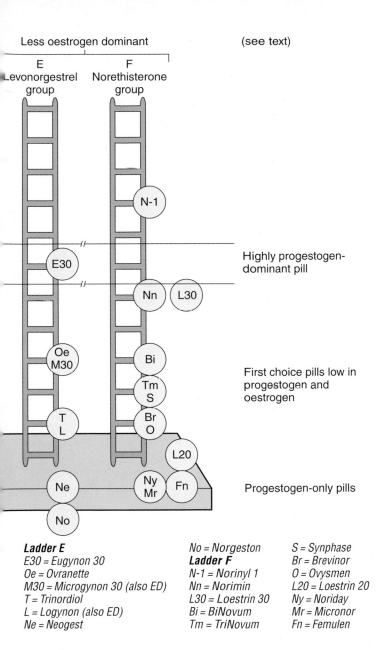

Less oestrogen dominant   (see text)

| E | F |
| Levonorgestrel group | Norethisterone group |

N-1

E30

Highly progestogen-dominant pill

Nn   L30

Oe M30   Bi

Tm S

First choice pills low in progestogen and oestrogen

T L   Br O

L20

Ne   Ny Mr   Fn

Progestogen-only pills

No

Ladder E
E30 = Eugynon 30
Oe = Ovranette
M30 = Microgynon 30 (also ED)
T = Trinordiol
L = Logynon (also ED)
Ne = Neogest

No = Norgeston
Ladder F
N-1 = Norinyl 1
Nn = Norimin
L30 = Loestrin 30
Bi = BiNovum
Tm = TriNovum

S = Synphase
Br = Brevinor
O = Ovysmen
L20 = Loestrin 20
Ny = Noriday
Mr = Micronor
Fn = Femulen

scientifically more valid. This is because the *different* progestogen is really LNG, which behaves anti-oestrogenically in many of its biological effects.

We have known for years that LNG tends to oppose the oestrogen-mediated rise in sex-hormone-binding globulin (SHBG) and high-density lipoprotein (HDL) cholesterol (and even lowers the latter if enough is given, see Figure 6). Somatically, it also opposes the tendency for oestrogen to improve acne. It is thus unlike most of the other marketed progestogens, which basically allow oestrogen to 'do its own thing'. A major study at the MPC compared the four main progestogens (DSG, GSD, LNG and NET) combined with the same 30 μg dose of EE. We confirmed (*without any assumptions about whether they are good or bad for health*) these biochemical differences between the two types of progestogen and the fact that NET is similar to, but less potent than, LNG in opposing at least some oestrogenic effects.

Does this mean a similar lessening by LNG and NET of oestrogen-mediated prothrombotic changes? The answer appears to be yes. New data from researchers in the Netherlands and the UK have now identified reduced effects of EE, if combined with LNG, on two such, namely acquired activated protein-C resistance and reduction of protein-S levels. Hence it is no longer biologically implausible that the combination of LNG with EE reduces the prothrombotic (oestrogenic) effects of EE below what they would be with a given dose of EE alone. It looks as though DSG and GSD and the other progestogens simply fail to have that opposing action, just as they do when we actually want a greater oestrogenic effect (e.g. when choosing a pill for someone with acne).

However, any beneficial effect of LNG and NET on VTE risk may not be as great as the epidemiology of 1995–1996 suggested. This is because of the well-

A) SHBG increment

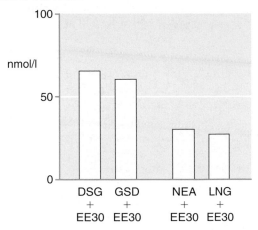

B) HDL cholesterol changes

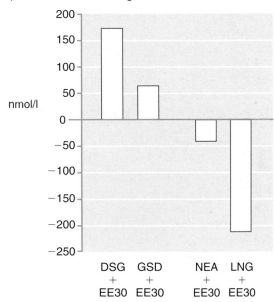

Figure 6
A) Prospective RCT of 4 pills: SHBG increment (MPC). B) Prospective RCT of 4 pills:
HDL cholesterol changes (MPC) See text

established influence of prescriber bias and the so-called healthy-user effect (leading at the time of the studies to LNG/NET pill use being more probable in women at lower intrinsic risk).

The advice in a press release (7 April 1999) from the Department of Health (DoH), issued after the 1998 review by the Medicines Commission of the VTE issue raised by the CSM in October 1995, still provides a good bottom line with regard to the COC and this one condition. They 'found no new safety concerns' about third-generation DSG or GSD products.

*An increased risk of venous thromboembolic disease (VTE) associated with the use of oral contraceptives is well established but is smaller than that associated with pregnancy; which has been estimated at 60 cases per 100 000 pregnancies. Some epidemiological studies have reported a greater risk of VTE for women using combined oral contraceptives containing desogestrel or gestodene (the so-called third generation pills) than for women using pills containing levonorgestrel (LNG) – the so-called second generation pills: (*Sic: category also includes NET pills*). The spontaneous incidence of VTE in healthy non-pregnant women (not taking any oral contraceptive) is about 5 cases per 100 000 women per year. The incidence in users of second generation pills is about 15 per 100 000 women per year of use. The incidence in users of third generation pills is about 25 cases per 100 000 women per year of use: <u>this excess incidence has not been satisfactorily explained by bias or confounding</u>. The level of all of these risks of VTE increases with age and is likely to be increased in women with other known risk factors for VTE such as obesity.*

Women must be fully informed of these very small risks ... Provided they are, the type of pill is for the woman together with her doctor or other family

planning professionals jointly to decide in the light of her individual medical history. [Author's emphasis.]

DoH, 7 April 1999

The underlined part of the above statement, and the levels of the absolute rates of VTE, are still disputed by some authorities, and by the manufacturers of DSG and GSD products. Even if the whole difference is accepted as real, Table 4 and Figure 7, where the denominator is per million rather than per 100 000, help to put the risks into perspective:

Table 4
Comparative risks – estimates 2004.

Annual risks per 1 000 000 women		
Activity	**Cases**	**Deaths**
Having a baby, UK (all direct causes of death)		60
Having a baby (VTE)	600	20
Using DSG/GSD pill (VTE)	250	5
Using LNG/NET pill (VTE)	150	3
Non-user, non-pregnant (VTE)	50–100	1–2
Risk from **all causes** through COC (healthy non-smoking woman)		10
Home accidents		30
Playing soccer		40
Road accidents		80
Parachuting (10 jumps/year)		200
Scuba diving		220
Hang-gliding		1500
Cigarette smoking (in next year if aged 35)		1670
Death from pregnancy/ childbirth in rural Africa		10 000 plus

Sources: Dinman BD (1980) *JAMA* **244**: 1226–8; Mills A et al (1996) *BMJ* **312**: 121; Anon (1991) *BMJ* **302**: 743; Strom B (1994) *Pharmacoepidemiology* 2nd edn (Chichester: Wiley) 57–65; www.doh.gov.uk/cmo/mdeaths.htm.

Note: VTE mortality assumed to be 2%; but higher in relation to pregnancy.

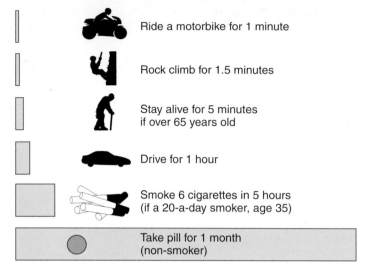

Ride a motorbike for 1 minute

Rock climb for 1.5 minutes

Stay alive for 5 minutes
if over 65 years old

Drive for 1 hour

Smoke 6 cigarettes in 5 hours
(if a 20-a-day smoker, age 35)

Take pill for 1 month
(non-smoker)

Time

Figure 7
Time required to have a 1:1 000 000 risk of dying. (Adapted from Minerva, British
Medical Journal, *1988.)*

Using the incidence rates given by the DoH above, each year there will be 100 fewer cases of VTE per million users of an LNG product such as Microgynon 30™ (Schering Health Care) than of a more oestrogen-dominant product. Using the high estimate of 2% for VTE mortality in the UK, this means only a 2 per million difference in annual VTE mortality between an oestrogen-dominant product and say Microgynon 30. From Figure 7, this risk difference is the same as that from 2 hours of driving. Hence, if a woman chooses (as she might very reasonably do after counselling), to control a side effect by switching away from Microgynon 30 to such a product: all she needs to do is avoid one 2-hour drive in the whole of the next year to remain, in terms of VTE risk, effectively still on the Microgynon 30!

Arterial wall disease

Does the apparent 'biological oestrogenicity' of DSG/GSD pills make them relatively better than LNG/NET pills for arterial wall diseases, especially acute myocardial infarction (AMI)? The epidemiology to date indicates that if there is an arterial wall advantage through taking DSG/GSD pills, it can only exist among Pill-takers with arterial risk factors such as smoking, since in their absence there **is** no arterial risk from the COC (see pp. 33–6.)

Prescribing guidelines
Which women are best for the Pill method?

'Current scientific evidence suggests only two prerequisites for the safe provision of COCs: a careful personal and family history with particular attention to cardiovascular risk factors, and a well-taken blood pressure' [Hannaford P, Webb A (1996). Evidence-guided prescribing of combined oral contraceptives: consensus statement. *Contraception* **54**: 125–9]. Therefore:

- Prescribers should always take a comprehensive personal and family history to exclude **absolute and relative contraindications** to the use of COCs (see Boxes on pp. 38–40). A personal history of definite VTE remains an absolute contraindication to any combined hormonal method [including EVRA™ or NuvaRing™] containing EE combined with any progestogen
2. The risk factors for VTE and arterial wall disease must be assessed separately and most carefully (see Tables 5 and 6). In this edition these are now classified according to the WHO eligibility criteria (see p. 8). Alone, one risk factor from either Table 5 or 6 is a relative contraindication (WHO 2 or 3 columns), unless it is particularly severe (WHO 4 column). Synergism means that if WHO 3 already applies, any additional risk factor moves the category to WHO 4 ('Do not use'). Generally, however, COC use is accceptable (WHO 3) when two WHO 2 factors apply. The remarks and footnotes in Tables 5 and 6 are fundamental to Pill prescribing.

Table 5
Risk factors for venous thromboembolism (VTE).

Risk factor	Absolute contraindication WHO 4	Relative contraindication WHO 3	Relative contraindication WHO 2	Remarks
FH of thrombophilia **or** of venous thrombosis in sibling or parent	Identified clotting abnormality of any kind (including acquired type) FH of a defined thrombophilia **or** idiopathic thrombotic event in parent or sibling < 45 and thrombophilia screen not (yet) available	FH of thrombosis in parent or sibling <45 with recognized precipitating factor, e.g. major surgery, post-partum and thrombophilia screen not available	FH of thrombotic event in parent or sibling <45 *with* or *without* a recognized precipitating factor and **Normal** thrombophilia screen FH in parent or sibling ≥45 **or** FH in 2nd degree relative (Classified WHO 2 but tests not indicated)	Idiopathic VTE in a parent or sibling <45 is an indication for a thrombophilia screen if available. The decision to undertake screening in other situations (including where there **was** a recognized precipitating factor), should be unusual as not cost effective – might be done on clinical grounds, in discussion with the woman Even a normal thrombophilia screen cannot be entirely reassuring (see text)
Overweight (high BMI)	BMI >39	BMI 30–39	BMI 25–29	
Immobility	Bed-bound **or** leg fractured and immobilized	Wheelchair life	Reduced mobility for other reason	

Table 5
continued

Risk factor	Absolute contraindication WHO 4	Relative contraindication WHO 3	Relative contraindication WHO 2	Remarks
VVs	Current superficial vein thrombosis in the upper thigh Current sclerotherapy for VVs	History of superficial vein thrombosis in the lower limbs, no deep vein thrombosis	–	Superficial vein thrombosis itself does not result in pulmonary embolism, though this past history is a reason for caution (WHO 3) in case it is a marker of future VTE risk (not confirmed). Exceptionally thrombosis of the greater saphenous vein in the thigh, reaching to the sapheno-femoral vein junction, may extend into the deep system – a history of such extension is WHO 4 for the COC
Age >35	Age >51	Age 35–51		

Notes

1. A single risk factor in relative contraindication column indicates use of LNG/NET pill if any COC used (see BNF).
2. N.B. synergism: more than one factor in either relative contraindication column. As a working rule, two WHO 2 conditions makes WHO 3; and if WHO 3 applies, addition of either a WHO 2 or WHO 3 condition normally means WHO 4 (do not use).
3. The literature on the association of smoking with VTE disease offers no consensus (compare arterial disease).
4. Acquired predispositions also exist through disease (see text in the list of absolute contraindications).
5. There are also important acute VTE risk factors, that need to be considered in individual cases: notably major or leg surgery, long-haul flights and dehydration through any cause.

Hereditary predispositions to VTE (thrombophilias)

Blanket screening by any blood test is not justifiable – not only would the cost be prohibitive but in terms of the occurrence of actual disease events there are just too many false negatives and positives. Almost the only indication for screening is a strong family history of one or more siblings or parents having had a spontaneous VTE under the age of 45. This justifies testing for the genetic predispositions, including Factor V Leiden (the genetic cause of activated protein-C resistance). Even if all the results are normal, the COC remains WHO 2. The woman cannot be totally reassured, since by no means all the predisposing abnormalities of the complex haemostatic system have yet been characterized. Such an individual, like any Pill-taker with one VTE-linked relative contraindication (3rd or 4th columns of Table 5), should normally receive a LNG/NET Pill, unless there is a clear *therapeutic indication* for COC therapy, in which case extra therapeutic benefits may be judged to outweigh any expected extra risks.

Acquired predispositions to VTE (thrombophilias)

Antiphospholipid antibodies which increase both VTE and arterial disease risk (Table 6, Note 4) may appear in a number of connective tissue disorders, most commonly in systemic lupus erythematosus (SLE). If identified, they absolutely contraindicate COC use (WHO 4).

Which pills are the current 'best buys' for women?

- First, *all marketed pills may now be considered first line* (see bold section in DoH statement on p. 26). Given the tiny possible difference in VTE mortality between the two 'generations', the woman's own choice of a DSG or GSD or other oestrogen-dominant product after (well-documented) discussion must be respected, even if based on no more than the presence of significant acne, a friend's recommendation or the need for better cycle control. If side effects (pp. 49–50) appear with a LNG or NET product initially or at any later stage, 'the informed user should be the chooser'
- *Young first-time users:* despite what has just been said, a low-dose LNG or NET product should, in my view, remain the *usual* first choice. This is because they will include an unknown subgroup who are VTE predisposed, VTE being a more relevant consideration than arterial disease at this age, and the pills suit the majority and cost less. (Consider also use of an ED pill-type, see Figure 11).
- *In the presence of a single WHO 2 or 3 risk factor for venous thrombosis:* the new Summary of Product Characteristics (SPCs) (data sheets) for COCs state that DSG/GSD products are contraindicated (WHO 4). I would agree that a LNG or NET product is certainly preferred if COC is used **for contraception**. If used for **therapy**, a different risk–benefit balance may apply: e.g. a woman with a BMI of 31 who, because of having severe acne with or without polycystic ovarian syndrome might use Marvelon 30 Yasmin™ or Dianette™ on a WHO 3 basis. (In my view, these all share the same oestrogen-dominant category, but only because they lack LNG: with its specific effects antagonizing EE – see pp. 24–5)
- *Women with a single definite arterial risk factor* (Table 6) – usually after a number of years VTE-free use *or* if the COC is used at all by a healthy and risk-factor-free woman above the age of 35 – changing to a DSG or GSD product might be (at least) discussed. Any advantages in so doing are far from established (p. 36). *The primary reason for ever changing brands is the control of side effects*

In premenopausal women AMI is almost exclusively a disease of *smokers*. No study, and there have been at least six good ones (including RCGP, Oxford/FPA, US Nurses and WHO), has been able to detect an increased risk of AMI in current or past pill-taking *non-smokers*. The available evidence is similar for haemorrhagic strokes. Ischaemic strokes are different: there is a small increased odds ratio of 1.5–2 from COC use alone. Hopefully this is

Table 6
Risk factors for arterial cardiovascular system disease.

Risk factor	Absolute contraindication WHO 4	Relative contraindication WHO 3	Relative contraindication WHO 2	Remarks
FH of atherogenic lipid disorder **or** of arterial CVS event in sibling or parent	Identified atherogenic lipid profile FH of a known atherogenic lipid disorder **or** idiopathic arterial event in sibling or parent <45 and lipid screening not (yet) available	FH of known lipid disorder or idiopathic arterial event in parent or sibling <45 and client's lipid profile 'borderline' atherogenic	FH of arterial event with risk factor (e.g. smoking) in parent or sibling <45 and lipid screen not available FH of idiopathic event in parent or sibling ≥45 **or** FH in 2nd degree relative [classified WHO 2 but tests not indicated]	Arterial CVS disease without other risk factors, or a known atherogenic lipid disorder in a parent or sibling <45 is an indication for a fasting lipid screen, if available. The decision to undertake a lipid screen in other situations (especially if there **was** a recognized precipitating risk factor e.g., smoking) is unlikely to be cost effective, but may be done on clinical grounds, in discussion with the woman. Despite any FH, normal lipid screen for an individual **is** reassuring, and means WHO 1 (contrasts with thrombophilia screens, Table 5) Check with laboratory as to the clinical significance of abnormal results for fasting lipids

Notes
1. Synergism: more than one factor in either relative contraindication column. As a working rule, two WHO 2 conditions makes WHO 3; and if WHO 3 applies, addition of either a WHO 2 or WHO 3 condition normally means WHO 4 ('Do not use').
2. The Pill seems to give no added adverse effect in arterial disease unless there is a risk factor. In continuing smokers, COC is generally stopped at the age of 35 in the UK. But WHO's Eligibility Criteria surprisingly permit the category WHO 3 above the age of 35 for smokers if <15 per day.
3. Note overweight appears in both Tables 5 and 6: if that is the sole risk factor it indicates use of a LNG/NET. pill (i.e. Table 5 takes precedence).
4. Antiphospholipid antibodies, if known to have been acquired, are WHO 4 on arterial as well as venous grounds (see text).

Table 6
Continued.

Risk factor	Absolute contraindication WHO 4	Relative contraindication WHO 3	Relative contraindication WHO 2	Remarks
Cigarette Smoking	≥40 cigarettes/day	15–39 cigarettes/day	<15 cigarettes/day	Cut-offs are a bit arbitrary
Diabetes Mellitus	Severe or diabetic complications present (e.g. retinopathy, renal damage)	Not severe/labile and no complications, young patient with short duration of DM		DM is always at least WHO 3 (safer options available)
Hypertension	BP≥160/100 mmHg on repeated testing	BP 140–159/90–99 mmHg	BP <140/90	These levels are in accordance with the British Hypertension Society and WHO
		On treatment for essential hypertension (well controlled)	Past toxaemia of pregnancy	See p.42 re toxaemia history as a risk factor
Overweight	BMI >39	BMI 30–39	BMI 25–29	
Migraine	Migraine with aura			
	Migraine without aura if severe prolonged attacks (>72 hours) or ergotamine-treated	Migraine without aura plus single WHO 2 arterial risk factor	Migraine without aura	Relates to stroke risk, see text
				Triptan treatment does not affect the category
Age >35	Age >51 (safer options available)	Age >40 in ex-heavy smokers to age 35	Age 35–51 in non-smokers	In ex-heavy smokers, the category WHO 3 (caution) above the age of 40 relates to possible persistence of earlier arterial wall damage

5. Some of the numbers selected are arbitrary and perhaps too strict if they are the sole problem (e.g. the COC might actually be allowed, reluctantly, to an otherwise currently healthy 25-year-old woman admitting to 40 cigarettes per day).

6. Numbers also relate to use for contraception: use of COCs for medical indications often entails a different risk-benefit analysis, i.e. the extra therapeutic benefits may outweigh expected extra risks. This point applies also to the conditions in Table 5.

further reducible by careful prescribing in *migraine* – see below.

So, the arterial event risk of using **all** the modern low-oestrogen brands must be very small if not absent for women free of arterial risk factors. However, the risk is high when such risk factors are present (the RCGP's relative risk estimate for AMI was 20.8 for smoking Pill-takers) and increases with age (see Table 6). Moreover the case-fatality rate for AMI in Pill-takers is also higher. Thus, I feel that we should not discount the suggestive evidence that DSG/GSD pills might have relative advantages for arterial wall disease, *but only in higher risk women.*

Therefore, switching to a low-oestrogen DSG or GSD Pill may reasonably be *discussed* with women who have any significant arterial risk factor *as they get older (assuming they do not accept a different method)*, for two reasons:

- It is only in the older age group that arterial disease becomes common enough to be relevant to prescribing policy;
- Any woman who has by then been on any combined pill – EE combined with any progestogen – for some years and/or has had a full-term pregnancy, is a 'survivor', i.e. relatively unlikely now to get VTE (not that this previous uncomplicated use eliminates that risk).

Femodette™ (Schering Health Care) (GSD) or Mercilon™ (Organon Laboratories) (DSG) are the 20 µg EE products which are my own usual suggestion for these women (*no later than 35 years of age*); and also in general for arterial risk factor-free women aged 35–51. Loestrin 20™ (Parke-Davis Medical) would also be acceptable, and better if there is any special concern about VTE risk.

Documentation
If a DSG/GSD pill is chosen, whether for this indication or

more often just because the woman prefers it on quality-of-life or side-effect grounds, there must be a full contemporaneous record:

- of the risk-factor history;
- that the woman accepts a possibly increased risk of VTE relative to other formulations, which can be usefully explained as 2 hours of driving per year (see p. 28).

Norgestimate, the progestogen in Cilest

Initially there were no good epidemiological data, so the CSM letter in 1995 left prescribing practice unchanged for this product. It is a fact that 20% of norgestimate ingested actually becomes LNG by metabolism. Thus, all Cilest users actually finish up with a pill that effectively delivers about 55 µg of LNG. This, if the above thinking is correct, may provide some counteraction of the oestrogenicity (and any prothrombogenicity) of the EE in Cilest.

In practice, pending more data, Cilest and the derived transdermal product EVRA, (see pp. 69–70), seem to be working out as slightly oestrogen-dominant middle-of-the-road compounds: useful for *many* women, but not especially for selection when one has a specific concern either about VTE or to provide a more oestrogenic effect.

Absolute contraindications to combined oral contraceptives (COCs)

All contraindications below are WHO 4. However, for the same conditions, POPs, including Cerazette and other progestogen-only methods, are in general only WHO 2 at most.

COCs – all brands (and EVRA) – are absolutely contraindicated in:

1. Past or present circulatory disease
- Any past proven arterial or venous thrombosis
- Ischaemic heart disease or angina or coronary arteritis (Kawasaki disease – but WHO 3 after full recovery)
- Severe or combined risk factors for venous or arterial disease (see Tables 5 and 6)
- Atherogenic lipid disorders (take advice from an expert, as indicated)
- Known prothrombotic abnormality of coagulation/fibrinolysis, i.e. congenital or acquired thrombophilias (p. 32); from at least 2 (preferably 4) weeks before until 2 weeks after mobilization following elective major or leg surgery (do not demand that the COC be stopped for minor surgery such as laparoscopy); during leg immobilization (e.g. after fracture or varicose vein treatment); and when going to high altitudes if there are added risk factors-otherwise WHO 3 (see below).
- Migraine with aura, (described on pp. 42–5)
- Transient ischaemic attacks and definite aura without headache following
- Past cerebral haemorrhage
- Pulmonary hypertension, any cause.
- Structural uncorrected heart disease such as *valvular heart disease or shunts/septal defects* are only WHO 4 if there is an added arterial or venous thromboembolic risk (persisting, if there has been surgery). Always discuss this with the cardiologist – could be WHO 3, especially if on warfarin. Important WHO 4 examples are atrial fibrillation or flutter whether sustained or paroxysmal or not current but high risk (e.g. mitral stenosis); dilated left atrium (more than 4 cm); cyanotic heart disease; any dilated cardiomyopathy but not a past history of any type when in full remission (WHO 2).
  In other structural heart conditions, if there is little or no direct or indirect risk of thromboembolism (this being *the* point to check with the cardiologist), the COC is usable (WHO 3 or 2)

2. Disease of the liver
- Active liver disease (whenever liver function tests currently abnormal, including infiltrations and cirrhosis); past Pill-related cholestatic jaundice (if in pregnancy can be WHO 3); Dubin–Johnson and Rotor syndromes (Gilbert's disease is WHO 2). Following viral hepatitis or other liver cell damage COCs may be resumed 3 months after liver function tests have become normal
- Liver adenoma, carcinoma
- Acute hepatic porphyrias; others are usually WHO 3, but a non-steroid hormone method usually preferable

Note that several of the above (e.g. 4–5, 8) are not necessarily permanent contraindications. Over the years many women have been unnecessarily deprived of COCs for reasons now shown to have no link, such as thrush, or which would have positively benefited from the method, such as secondary amenorrhoea with hypo-oestrogenism.

Relative contraindications to combined oral contraceptives (COCs)

Using WHO's scheme, but categorised according to my judgement of the evidence, below are listed the relative contraindications to COCs, signifying that the COC method is usable in context with:

- the benefit–risk evaluation for that individual;
- the acceptability or otherwise of alternatives;
- sometimes with special advice (e.g. in migraine, to report a change of symptomatology) or monitoring.

In cases with excess risk of venous thrombosis (e.g. wheelchair life), if the Pill is used at all for contraception it should be a LNG/NET variety.

Relative contraindications to COCs (WHO 2 unless otherwise stated).

- Risk factors for arterial or venous disease (*see* Tables 5 and 6): these are WHO 3, sometimes 2, provided that only one is present and not to such a degree as to justify WHO 4; for diabetes, essential hypertension, pregnancy toxaemia and migraine see pp. 41–5
- Risk of altitude illness. This is not caused by COC, but in its most severe forms there may be venous or arterial thromboembolism or patchy pulmonary hypertension, which of course contraindicate the method. All women travelling to above 2500 m should be informed that the COC might minimally increase such risk and will be intrinsic in their particular exposure to high altitude. The COC would be WHO 3, in general, but could be only WHO 2 in many healthy trekkers who intend always to follow the maxim 'climb high but sleep low'. More details in BMJ 2003; 326: 915–19.
- Sex-steroid-dependent cancer (e.g. breast cancer) in prolonged remission (WHO 3): the latter is defined as 5 years by WHO (Melanoma is WHO 2 for the Pill)
- If a young (less than 40 years of age), first-degree relative has breast cancer (WHO 2)
- Established benign breast disease (if with atypia is WHO 4; p. 15)
- During the monitoring of *abnormal cervical smears* (WHO 2)
- During and after definitive *treatment for CIN* (WHO 2)
- Oligo-/amenorrhoea (COCs may be prescribed after investigation – may even be WHO 1 if used to supply oestrogen in a woman needing contraception or to control the symptoms of PCOS)
- Hyperprolactinaemia (relative contraindication WHO 3 for patients under specialist drug treatment and supervision)
- Most chronic congenital or acquired diseases (see p. 41) are WHO 2; homozygous sickle cell disease WHO 2, though DMPA even better (p. 85) (sickle cell trait is WHO 1); inflammatory bowel disease WHO 2, or 3 if severe because of VTE risk in exacerbations; otosclerosis (WHO 2)
- HUS may be WHO 3 if complete recovery and not Pill associated (e.g. past E coli 0157 infection as cause of HUS).
- Gallstones (WHO 3, but WHO 2 after cholecystectomy)
- Diseases that require long-term treatment with enzyme-inducing drugs (see pp. 60–4) are WHO 3
- Very severe depression, if likely to be exacerbated by COCs (but unwanted pregnancies can be very depressing!

Intercurrent diseases

It is impossible for the Boxes immediately above to list every known disease which might have a bearing (i.e. WHO 4, 3 or 2) on COC prescription, and for many the data are unavailable. A working rule therefore is to ascertain whether or not the condition might lead to **summation** with known major adverse effects of COCs, particularly with the risk of any circulatory disease; this usually means WHO 4, sometimes 3. If it won't summate, in most serious chronic conditions the patient can be reassured that COCs are not known to have any effect, good or bad; they may then be used (WHO 2), though with the most careful monitoring and alertness for the onset of new risk factors. Reliable protection from pregnancy is often particularly important when other diseases are present, though we do now have new EE-free choices (e.g. Cerazette, Implanon, IUDs and the IUS).

Diabetes (generally a WHO 3 condition)

Mercilon or Femodette (see p. 36) can be valuable for limited periods, under careful supervision and provided that there is no arteriopathy, retinopathy, neuropathy or renal damage (or obesity or smoking!) – all of which mean WHO 4 – and preferably if the duration of the diabetes has been short (Table 6).

The POP (often Cerazette) or Implanon are good alternative options in the young; with perhaps a modern copper IUD, the LNG IUS or sterilization to follow later.

Hypertension

Hypertension is an important risk factor for both heart disease and stroke (see Table 6 and pp. 53 and 54).

- In most women on COCs there is a slight increase in both systolic and diastolic BP within the normotensive range: approximately 1% become clinically hypertensive (WHO 4 for the Pill, if clearly Pill–induced) and the rate increases with age and duration of use
- Past severe toxaemia (pregnancy-induced hypertension) does not predispose to hypertension during COC use but it is a risk factor for myocardial infarction (WHO 2), markedly so if the women also smokes (WHO 3)
- Essential hypertension (which is not COC related), when well controlled on drugs, is WHO 3.

Migraine

Like hypertension, this condition is important both at the first prescription and during the follow-up of Pill-takers. Migraines can be defined as unpleasant headaches which 'stop the person doing things' – usually one-sided, accompanied by nausea and/or photophobia/phonophobia.

- Studies have shown an increased risk of ischaemic stroke in migraine sufferers and in COC-users
- There is good evidence of exacerbation of this risk by arterial risk factors, including smoking and increasing age above 35 years
- Certain features of the headaches tend to focus the stroke risk – above all, the presence of aura before the headache (see Table 6 and Figure 8).

Migraine with aura

Timing is crucial: *neurological symptoms of aura begin before the headache itself*, and typically last around 20–30 minutes. Headache may start as aura resolves or there may first be a gap of up to 1 hour.

- Visual symptoms occur in 99% of true auras:
  - these are typically bright and affect part of the **field** of vision, on the same side in both eyes (homonymous hemianopia)
  - teichopsia/fortification spectra are often described, typically a bright scintillating zig-zag line gradually enlarging from a bright centre on one side, to form a convex C-shape surrounding the area of lost vision (a *bright* scotoma)
- Sensory symptoms are confirmatory of aura, occurring in around one third of cases and rarely in the absence of visual aura. Typically they come as 'pins and needles' (paraesthesia) spreading up one arm or one side of the face or the tongue; the leg is rarely affected
- Disturbance of speech (usually nominal dysphasia)

Note the absence in the above box of the symptoms which occur during headache itself (photophobia or *generalized* blurring or 'flashing lights'). Aura symptoms should not be confused with *premonitory symptoms,* such as food cravings, extra sensitivity to light and sound, occurring up to a day or two before any migraine (i.e. with or without aura).

Taking an aura history.
- Ask the woman to describe a typical attack from the very beginning, including any symptoms before a headache. Listen to what she says *but at the same time watch her carefully*
- A most useful **SIGN** that it is likely to be true aura is if, when asked to describe what she sees, she draws a zig-zag line in the air with a finger to one or other side of her own head

Absolute contraindications (WHO 4) to starting or continuing the COC.
- *Migraine with aura during which there are the above neurological symptoms.* The *artificial oestrogen* of the COC is what needs to be avoided (or stopped) to minimize the additional risk of a thrombotic stroke. Rarely, aura occurs without headache (still WHO 4).
- *All other migraines (even without aura) which are exceptionally severe during Pill taking* and last more than 72 hours
- *All migraines treated with ergot derivatives*, due to their vasoconstrictor actions
- *Migraine without aura occurring during Pill taking* **plus** two or more additional arterial risk factors from Table 6, or relevant interacting diseases (e.g. connective tissue diseases linked with stroke risk)

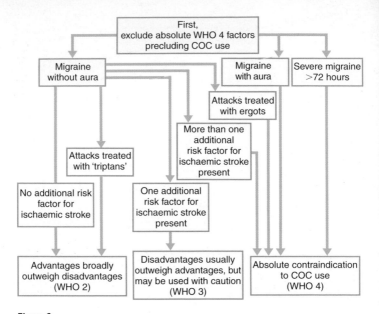

Figure 8
Flow diagram for COC use and migraine. (Reproduced from MacGregor A, Guillebaud J (1998) Br J Family Planning 24: 53–60.)

In all the above circumstances any of the *progestogen-only*, i.e. *oestrogen-free* hormonal methods may be offered immediately. Similar headaches may continue but without the potential added risk from prothrombotic effects of EE. Particularly useful choices are Cerazette, Implanon and the LNG IUS, or a modern copper IUD.

Migraine: relative contraindications (WHO 3 or 2) for the COC. WHO 3
- **Primarily**, this is migraine without aura (common/simple migraine) where one WHO 2 (not severe) risk factor for ischaemic stroke is present (see Figure 8). A good example is age above 35.
- **Secondly**, a clear past history of typical migraine *with aura* more than 5 years earlier or only during pregnancy, with no recurrence, may be regarded as WHO 3. COCs may be given a trial, with

counselling and regular supervision, along with a specific warning that the onset of definite aura (carefully explained) means that the user should

- stop the Pill immediately
- use alternative contraception and
- seek medical advice as soon as possible

WHO 2 In my opinion the COC is 'Broadly usable' in all the following cases:

- *Migraine without aura*, and also without any arterial risk factor from Table 6 and still under the age of 35. NB: If these (or other 'ordinary' headaches) occur only or mainly in the pill-free interval (PFI), tricycling the COC may help
- *Use of a triptan drug* in the absence of any other contraindicating factors.
- *The occurrence of a woman's first-ever attack of migraine without aura while on the COC.* It is a reasonable precaution to stop the Pill if she is seen during the attack. But after full evaluation of the symptoms – provided there were no features of aura or marked risk factors – the COC can be later restarted (WHO 2), with the usual counselling/caveats about future aura

The attributable risk rises with age. According to Lidegaard's data from Denmark in the early 1990s (in which subjects had migraine of some kind occurring at least once per month), the background annual risk of thrombotic stroke for women at 20 years of age is 2 in 100 000. With migraine at least once per month, plus taking COC, this rises to 10 in 100 000. But at 40 years of age background risk is 20 in 100 000, rising to 56 with migraine (same attack frequency). With the same relative risk (1.8) as found for younger women, adding the COC makes 100 in 100 000 total incidence! And that is without being able to quantify the extra risk of focal aura.

Counselling and ongoing supervision

Starting the COC (Table 7)

Each woman needs individual teaching, backed by the FPA's user-friendly leaflet *Your Guide to the Combined Pill*, which includes an important section (similar to that on

Table 7
Starting routines for combined oral contraceptives.

Conditions before start	Start when?	Extra precautions for 7 days
1. Menstruating	On day 1 or 2 of period	No*
	On day 3 or later	Yes*
	Any time in cycle (Quick Start)	Yes†
2. Postpartum (a) No lactation	Day 21‡ (low risk of thrombosis: first ovulations reported after day 28)	No
(b) Lactation	Not normally recommended (POP or injectable preferred)	
3. After induced abortion/miscarriage	Same day or day 2 (Day 21 if beyond 24 weeks gestation)	No
4. After trophoblastic tumour	One month after no hCG detected	As (1)
5. After higher dose COC	Instant switch or use condoms after PFI for 7 days§	No
6. After lower or same-dose COC	After usual 7-day break	No
7. After POP	First day of period	No*
8. During POP-induced secondary amenorrhoea	Any day (end of packet)	No
9. Other secondary amenorrhoea including after DMPA (pregnancy excluded)‖	Any day	Yes
10. First period after postcoital contraception	By day 2 when woman sure her flow is normal or Quick Start†, i.e. immediately (see p. 128)	No*

*Except some 28-day (ED) pills, where extra precautions recommended for 14 days. In the other situations here, start with the first *active* tablet.
†'Quick Start' refers to starting any day in selected cases, if the prescriber is satisfied there has been no risk of conception earlier, up to the starting day (see also p. 141).
‡Puerperal risk lasts longer after *severe* pregnancy-related hypertension, or the related HELLP (hypertension, elevated liver enzymes, low platelets) syndrome, so delay COC use until the return of normal BP and biochemistry. This history in the past is WHO 1.
§If usual 7-day break, rebound ovulation may occur at the time of transfer.
‖Meaning prescriber is confident that no blastocyst or sperm is already in the upper genital tract, if necessary through a negative sensitive pregnancy test after at least 14 days of safe contraception or abstinence from intercourse.

p. 53) listing the symptoms which should trigger taking urgent medical advice. This leaflet should always be given and its publication date noted in the patient's case notes. At the MPC it is also policy to check with all follow-up patients if they still have it. Table 7 gives the recommended starting routines. After dealing with the patient's concerns about risks, benefits and 'minor' side effects, the main take-home messages to be conveyed to a new user are highlighted on p. 68.

Second choice of pill brand

Some women react unpredictably and it is a false expectation that any single pill will suit all women. Individual variations in motivation and tolerance of minor side effects are well recognized. But, due to differences in absorption and metabolism, there is also marked variability (threefold, in the area under the curve) in *blood levels of the exogenous hormones* (Figure 9).

Bleeding side effects

Given the model provided in Figure 9, prescribers should try to identify the lowest dose for each woman which does

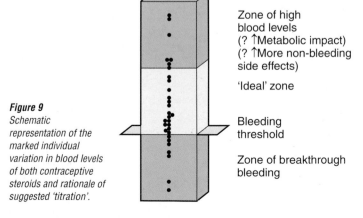

Figure 9
Schematic representation of the marked individual variation in blood levels of both contraceptive steroids and rationale of suggested 'titration'.

Zone of high blood levels
(? ↑Metabolic impact)
(? ↑More non-bleeding side effects)

'Ideal' zone

Bleeding threshold

Zone of breakthrough bleeding

not cause breakthrough bleeding (BTB). This should minimize adverse side effects, both serious and minor, and also reduce measurable metabolic changes. Since combined pills all have a powerful contraceptive effect, this approach does not appear to impair effectiveness (far more important is not lengthening the PFI; see pp. 54–9). Indeed, even if BTB occurs, extra contraception (e.g. with condoms) does not need to be advised, provided there is ongoing good compliance with Pill taking.

The objective is that each woman should receive the least long-term metabolic impact that her uterus will allow, i.e. the lowest dose of contraceptive steroids that is just, but only just, above her bleeding threshold. If there is good cycle control, therefore, and a lower dose brand in the same 'ladder' (Figure 5) is available, switching to it at an appropriate time should be considered.

What if BTB occurs and is unacceptable or persists beyond two cycles? A different or higher dose brand (Figure 5) should be tried, though only **after** the checks in the Box (p. 49). Phasic COCs are second-choice formulations in my own practice, but they are certainly worth trying here for BTB and especially for absence of withdrawal bleeding. If cycle control can only be achieved by a 50 or 60 µg oestrogen pill *combination*, this could rarely be justifiable with good counselling, monitoring and records (but check Tables 5 and 6 and the named-patient guidelines on p. 141). Note: In this respect Norinyl-1™ (Searle) differs little from Norimin™ (Searle) (see p. 63).

It is vital to exclude other causes of BTB before blaming the COC!

The following, very helpful, checklist has been modified from Sapire [*Contraception and Sexuality in Health and Disease*, New York: McGraw-Hill].

- **DISEASE** Examine the cervix (it is not unknown for bleeding from an invasive cancer to be wrongly attributed, and any bloodstained discharge should always trigger the thought '*Chlamydia?*')
- **DISORDERS of PREGNANCY** that cause bleeding (e.g. retained products if COC was started after a recent termination of pregnancy)
- **DEFAULT** (BTB may start 2 or 3 days after missed pills and may be persistent thereafter)
- **DRUGS**, primarily enzyme inducers (see text). Cigarettes have also been implicated: BTB is statistically more common among smokers
- **Diarrhoea** and/or **VOMITING** (diarrhoea alone has to be very severe to impair absorption significantly)
- **DISTURBANCES of ABSORPTION**, for example after massive gut resection (coeliac disease does not pose an absorption problem)
- **Diet** (the gut flora involved in recycling EE may be reduced in vegetarians, but this is a very unlikely cause)
- **DURATION of USE** too short – i.e. assessment is too early (minimal BTB which is tolerable for a bit longer may cease after 3 months use of any new formulation). The opposite possibility may apply during tricycling (see pp. 51–2), namely that the duration of continuous use has been too long for that woman's endometrium to be sustained, in which case a *bleeding–triggered* 4–7 day break may be taken; or bicycling of two packets in a row may be substituted
- **DOSE**, after the above have been excluded, it is possible to try a phasic pill if the woman is receiving monophasic treatment; increase the progestogen component (or oestrogen if Mercilon is in use); try a different progestogen; or consider a 50 or 60 μg pill combination (strictly on a named-patient basis, see text)

Second choice if there are non-bleeding side effects

When symptoms occur it is generally bad practice to give further prescriptions, such as diuretics for weight gain or antidepressants.

There are two main preferred, if empirical, courses of action: (1) to decrease the dose of either hormone, if still possible (in the limit, oestrogen can be eliminated by a trial of the POP); or (2) to change to a different progestogen. Although the evidence is mainly anecdotal, there is some specific guidance available for side effects and conditions associated with a relative excess of either steroid.

Which second choice of pill? Relative oestrogen excess.	
Symptoms	**Conditions**
• Nausea • Dizziness • Cyclical weight gain (fluid), 'bloating' • Vaginal discharge (no infection) • Some cases of breast enlargement/pain • Some cases of lost libido without depression, especially if taking an anti-androgen (Yasmin or Dianette)	• Benign breast disease • Fibroids • Endometriosis

Treat with progestogen-dominant COC, such as Microgynon 30, Loestrin 30 or Eugynon 30™ (Schering Health Care), (but with caution regarding lipids, and risk of arterial disease in those with the relevant risk factors, see pp. 33–6). Loestrin 20 and the new 20 mg EE+LNG pill are oestrogen-deficient options

Which second choice of pill? Relative progestogen excess.	
Symptoms	**Conditions**
• Dryness of vagina • Some cases of: Sustained weight gain Depression/lassitude Loss of libido with depressed mood Breast tenderness	• Acne/seborrhoea • Hirsutism

Treat with oestrogen-dominant COC, such as Marvelon™ (Organon Laboratories), Ovysmen™ (Janssen-Cilag)/Brevinor™ (Searle), or, in moderately severe cases of acne or hirsutism Yasmin or Dianette (see text). [Caution necessary in that oestrogen dominance may correlate with a slightly higher risk of VTE, especially in, for example obesity (Table 5)].

More about Yasmin
Acne, seborrhoea and sometimes hirsutism may be benefited by any of the oestrogen-dominant COCs, whereas there is less or no benefit when there is progestogen dominance.

Yasmin is a monophasic COC with 3.0 mg DSP and 30 µg EE. DSP differs from other progestogens in COCs because:

- it acts an anti-androgen, so the combination is an alternative to Dianette for the treatment of moderately severe acne and the PCOS;
- it has diuretic properties due to antimineralocorticoid activity.

Yasmin is welcomed as a new oestrogen-dominant choice for appropriate women. My own criteria for using it are as follows:

> - A clear indication for oestrogen/anti-androgen therapy
> - During COC follow-up, as a useful oestrogen-dominant second choice for empirical control of minor side effects: particularly those associated with fluid retention such as bloatedness and cyclical breast enlargement
> - Raised BP at a level suggesting a change from the current formulation but COC still clinically usable and much wanted by the woman, i.e. BP at or slightly above 140/90 mmHg which is the upper limit of WHO 2 for raised BP (Table 6). More research is needed on this possibility. A POP such as Cerazette would be a good alternative
> - Last, and definitely least, what about weight? In a study there was a maintained slight (about 1%) reduction of body mass, but probably due only to less total body water compared with controls. Also if the body mass index (BMI) is already above 30 there is a safety issue, and a less oestrogen-dominant formulation with LNG or NET should normally be chosen (pp. 32, 33). Otherwise *anxiety* about weight or a history of fluid retention-linked weight gain with earlier pills might rarely justify its use

Where does Dianette feature now?

This is another anti-androgen plus oestrogen combination (CPA 2 mg with EE 35 µg), licensed for the treatment of moderately severe acne and mild hirsutism in women. These are its indications, but practically everything about the COC in this book applies also to Dianette: it is a reliable anovulant, usually giving good cycle control, and has similar rules for missed tablets, interactions, absolute and relative contraindications, and requirements for monitoring.

There has been no good head-to-head randomized comparative trial (RCT) of Yasmin versus Dianette reported, but indirect evidence suggests that Yasmin would have at least as good effectiveness for the conditions for which Dianette is indicated, and so might usefully be used from the outset. Both are oestrogen-dominant products requiring careful assessment of VTE risk factors: an increased VTE risk compared with LNG pills has been shown for Dianette, but not so far for Yasmin.

Duration of treatment with Dianette needs to be individualized. In the SPC (data sheet) it is recommended that 'treatment is withdrawn when the acne or hirsutism is completely resolved', but 'repeat courses may be given if the condition recurs'. There are some concerns (not confirmed) related to hepatic effects, including of a greater benign and malignant liver tumour risk than other COCs in long-term use. So it is usual to encourage patients to switch when their condition is controllod, peihaps after about 1 year, commonly to Marvelon, which can be promoted to the woman as likely to be quite sufficient as *maintenance* treatment for (now) milder acne. If there is a relapse, try Yasmin; or exceptionally it may be appropriate to use Dianette for much longer.

Stopping COCs

The first menstruation after stopping COCs (for any reason) is often delayed by up to about 6–8 weeks. Secondary amenorrhoea for 6 months should always be investigated, whether or not it occurs after stopping COCs – the link is coincidental and not causal. Whatever the diagnosis, if there is associated oestrogen deficiency it should always be treated.

The Box below lists the (only) reasons for discontinuing COCs immediately or soon, and should be understood by all well-counselled women from their first visit. The worst implications of most of these symptoms are Pill-related thrombotic or embolic catastrophes in the making, but more often there is another explanation. They mean that EE should be stopped, but any POP method could be started immediately pending diagnosis. The symptoms appear in lay terms in the FPA's recommended leaflet *Your Guide to the Combined Pill*.

Symptoms for which COCs should be stopped immediately, pending investigation and treatment.
- Unusual or severe and very prolonged headache
- Diagnosis of aura, usually with loss of part or whole of the field of vision on one side, or loss of sight in one eye
- Disturbance of speech (nominal dysphasia)
- Numbness, severe paraesthesia or weakness on one side of the body, e.g. one arm, side of the tongue; indeed, any symptom suggesting cerebral ischaemia
- A severe unexplained fainting attack or severe acute vertigo or ataxia
- Focal epilepsy
- Painful swelling in the calf
- Pain in the chest, especially pleuritic pain
- Breathlessness or cough with bloodstained sputum
- Severe abdominal pain
- Immobilization, as after most lower limb fractures or *major* surgery or leg surgery: stop COC and consider heparin treatment. If elective procedure and pill stopped more than 2 weeks ahead (4 weeks preferable), anticoagulation may be unnecessary

Other reasons for early discontinuation:
- Acute jaundice
- BP above 160/100 mmHg on repeated measurement
- Severe skin rash (e.g. erythema multiforme)
- Detection of a significant new risk factor, e.g. onset of SLE, detection of breast cancer

---

Pill follow-up: What are the requirements for monitoring?

Aside from the management of important risk factors or diseases already present, or that may suddenly or more gradually appear, and of new minor side effects (both dealt with above), follow-up primarily entails monitoring:

- BP
- headaches, especially migraine;
- aspects of the PFI, with implications for efficacy, drug interactions and some side effects.

Note what is **not** included: breast and bimanual pelvic examinations have no relevance to pill follow-up, they should only be performed for a specific clinical indication.

Blood Pressure
Monitoring of BP is vital (pp. 41–2). It should be recorded before COCs are started and checked after 3 months (1 month in a high-risk case) and subsequently at intervals of 6 months. After a minimum of 15 months, the interval can reasonably be increased to annually in women without risk factors, if there is no rise between successive measurements. COCs should always be stopped altogether if BP exceeds 160/100 mmHg on repeated measurements. A more moderate increase still suggests the possibility of an increased risk of arterial disease, especially in the presence of any other arterial risk factors.

Headaches
For migraine and its implications see pp. 42–5.

The 'pill-free interval' (PFI)

As no contraceptive is being taken during the PFI, it has important efficacy implications (Figure 10). Biochemical and ultrasound data obtained at the MPC and elsewhere

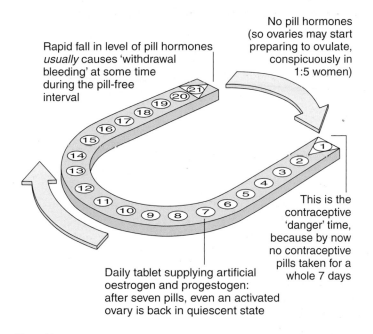

Rapid fall in level of pill hormones *usually* causes 'withdrawal bleeding' at some time during the pill-free interval

No pill hormones (so ovaries may start preparing to ovulate, conspicuously in 1:5 women)

This is the contraceptive 'danger' time, because by now no contraceptive pills taken for a whole 7 days

Daily tablet supplying artificial oestrogen and progestogen: after seven pills, even an activated ovary is back in quiescent state

Figure 10
'Horseshoe' analogy to explain the 21-day cycle. Omission of tablets either side of the gap in the horseshoe lengthens the "contraception-losing interval". See text.

demonstrate return of significant pituitary and ovarian follicular activity during the PFI in about 20% of cases – to a marked extent in some. Therefore, breakthrough ovulation is likely to follow any lengthening of the PFI. Figure 10 is a useful representation since the horseshoe is a symmetrical object. Lengthening of the PFI might be caused either side of the horseshoe; i.e. from omissions, malabsorption as from vomiting (an advantage of the new combined products EVRA and NuvaRing), or drug interactions involving pills either at the start or at the end of a packet.

In 1986, a population of current Pill-users was studied after the end of a routine PFI. The study showed that if only 14 or even as few as seven pills were then taken, no ovulation occurred after seven pills were subsequently missed. This implies at the very least that up to five pills may be missed mid-packet with impunity. This and other work may be summarized as follows:

> • seven consecutive pills are enough 'to shut the door' on the ovaries (therefore pills 8–21, or longer during tricycling, simply 'keep the door shut');
> • seven pills can be omitted without ovulation, as indeed is regularly the case in the PFI;
> • More than seven pills missed (*in total*) risks ovulation.

Based on this pharmacology, WHO has issued new advice for missed pills (see www.who.int/reproductive-health, click 'family planning' and go to 'selected practice recommendations'). I have modified this slightly (see Figure 11) to ensure that seven days of condom use is triggered early enough if the PFI is lengthened. One day late, making it 8 days in duration, risks ovulation in one of those highly susceptible 20%, during the next 7 days of pill taking. More than 24 hours late, or two or more pills missed in the first week, with ongoing sexual exposure indicates emergency contraception as well.

Note that in Figure 11 – rightly, in my view – this new policy removes the condom recommendation altogether in most circumstances where omissions occur in the second or third week of tablet taking. If 28-day packs are used, which I am sure help to avoid risky late restarts, the user must learn which are the dummy 'reminder' tablets. If she ever makes her own break prematurely – through missing some of the last seven active pills – these placebos must be omitted. Incidentally, if she does this, missing her next routine PFI, she will be even *less* likely to ovulate than usual. All women should be asked to report back if they have no bleeding in the *next* PFI.

Note also another major change by WHO, to make the trigger for any action being 1 day (i.e. 24 hours) late in pill

Every time you miss one or more active pills (days 1–21):

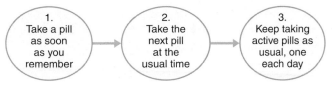

1.
Take a pill
as soon
as you
remember

2.
Take the
next pill
at the
usual time

3.
Keep taking
active pills as
usual, one
each day

In these special cases, ALSO follow these special rules:

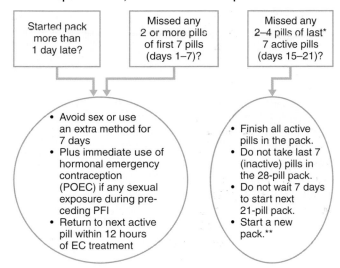

Started pack
more than
1 day late?

Missed any
2 or more pills
of first 7 pills
(days 1–7)?

Missed any
2–4 pills of last*
7 active pills
(days 15–21)?

- Avoid sex or use
  an extra method for
  7 days
- Plus immediate use of
  hormonal emergency
  contraception
  (POEC) if any sexual
  exposure during pre-
  ceding PFI
- Return to next active
  pill within 12 hours
  of EC treatment

- Finish all active
  pills in the pack.
- Do not take last 7
  (inactive) pills in
  the 28-pill pack.
- Do not wait 7 days
  to start next
  21-pill pack.
- Start a new
  pack.**

If you miss any of the 7 inactive pills (in a 28-pill* pack only):**

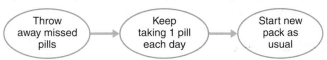

Throw
away missed
pills

Keep
taking 1 pill
each day

Start new
pack as
usual

Figure 11
Advice for missed pills (not more than 4 in number).
*For what to do if more than 4 pills are missed in days 8–21, see p. 129.
** 28-pill (ED) packs can obviously help some pill-takers not to forget to restart after each PFI (the contraception-losing interval). See p. 56. Even with triphasic pills, you should go straight to (the first phase of) the same brand. You may bleed a bit but you will still strengthen your contraception. This is quite different from postponing a 'period'. See p. 59.
*** 28-pill (ED) packs can obviously help some pill-takers not to forget to restart after each PFI (the contraception-losing interval). See p. 56.

taking, not the traditional 12 hours, which itself was never evidence based. I consider this acceptable, in the light of accumulated Pill studies over many years that demonstrate a considerably larger margin for error in pill taking than (even) 1 day.

Vomiting and diarrhoea

If vomiting began over 3 hours after one pill was taken, it can be assumed to have been absorbed. Otherwise follow Figure 11, according to the number and timing of the tablets deemed to have been missed. Diarrhoea alone is not a problem, unless it is of cholera-like severity.

Previous combined pill failure

Women who have had a previous COC failure may claim perfect compliance or perhaps admit to omission of no more than one pill. Either way, as surveys show, most women who miss a tablet quite frequently rarely conceive, so pill-failure tells us more about the individual's physiology than her memory. She is likely to be a member of that one fifth of the population whose ovaries show above average return to activity in the PFI. Such women may therefore be advised to take either three (Figure 12) or four packets in a row followed by a shortened PFI. Both these regimens are often termed *tricycling*. In the absence of dedicated packaging, 6 days is a possible choice for the PFI as it is easy to remember, the start day of each tricycle being identical to the weekday it finished.The gap is shortened further, usually to 4 days, in high conception-risk cases, such as during the use of enzyme inducers (see pp. 60–4).

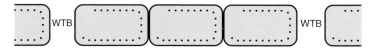

Figure 12
Tricycling (three or four-or more- packs in a row). Note that they must be monophasic packs.
Duration of PFI may also be shortened. WTB = withdrawal bleeds.

Once it has been appreciated that the Achilles heel of the COC is the PFI, the COC can always be made 'stronger' as a contraceptive, by eliminating and/or shortening the PFI through numerous variations on the tricycling theme depicted in Figure 12 (see also *bicycling*, below).

Why have PFIs at all?

The pill-free week does promote a reassuring withdrawal bleed (and, indeed, if this does not occur in two successive cycles it is best to eliminate pregnancy using a sensitive urine test). If this is not seen as important, and to obtain the other advantages, any woman may omit the PFIs and associated bleeds as a long-term *option*. Seasonale is a dedicated packaging in the USA which provides four packets of the formulation of Microgynon/ Ovranette™ (Wyeth Laboratories) in a row, followed by a 7-day, pill-free week, such that the user has a bleed every 3 months (i.e. seasonally!). This variant requires 16 packets a year as compared with usual 13 packs. Since for any given pill brand used this will obviously add to the annual ingested dose, it cannot be expected to reduce the risks of major or minor side effects: though the prospective user should be advised that there is also no evidence it will significantly increase them.

The gap between packets is often omitted in the short term (upon request) to avoid a 'period' on special occasions.* Longer term, in addition to the woman's choice, there exist some special indications, listed in the Box on p. 60, for using a tricycle regimen, which includes the option of taking a 20 µg brand like Loestrin 20* daily indefinitely, with no breaks.

---

* Users of phasic pills who wish to postpone withdrawal bleeds must use the final phase of a spare packet, or pills from an equivalent formulation, e.g. Norimin in the case of TriNovum™ (Janssen-Cilag) or Microgynon 30, immediately after the last tablet of Logynon™ (Schering Health Care).

BTB may occur during tricycling, implying that the Pill for that woman is unable to maintain endometrial stability for so long. One solution, provided a minimum of seven tablets have been taken since the last PFI (and it will usually be far more) is to advise at any time a definite 4–7 day break. This sometimes clears the decks so that the BTB stops once the next new cycle of tablets commences. Some women tolerate bicycling best, i.e. 42 days of continuous pill taking followed, depending on the indication, by a 4–7 day PFI.

Indications for a tricycling regimen (such as that shown in Figure 12) using a monophasic pill. In the last 3 instances (only), the PFI should be shortened to 4 days.
- Woman's choice
- Headaches, including migraine without aura and other bothersome symptoms if they occur regularly in the withdrawal week
- Unacceptably heavy or painful withdrawal bleeds
- Paradoxically, to help women who are concerned about absent withdrawal bleeds (less frequent pregnancy tests for reassurance!)
- Premenstrual syndrome – tricycling helps if COCs are used for this (p. 10)
- Endometriosis, where after primary therapy a progestogen-dominant monophasic pill may be tricycled for maintenance treatment
- Epilepsy, which benefits from relatively more sustained levels of the administered hormones, and tricycling with a shortened PFI may also be indicated by the therapy given
- Long term enzyme-inducer therapy (see p. 63–4)
- Wherever there is suspicion of decreased efficacy (see p. 58)

Drug interactions

Drug interactions reduce the efficacy of COCs mainly by induction of liver enzymes, which leads to increased elimination of both oestrogen and progestogen (Figure 13). Additionally, in a very small (but unknown) minority of women, disturbance by certain broad-spectrum antibiotics of the gut flora which normally split oestrogen metabolites that arrive in the bowel can reduce the reabsorption of reactivated oestrogen. This effect is not a factor in the

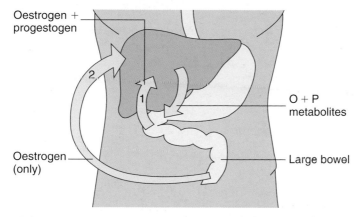

Figure 13
The enterohepatic recirculation of oestrogen.

maintenance of progestogen levels and so is irrelevant to the POP. The most clinically important drugs with which interaction occurs are given in the Boxes below.

Enzyme-inducer drugs (important examples) that interact with COCs.
- Rifampicin, rifabutin
- Griseofulvin (antifungal)
- Barbiturates
- Phenytoin
- Carbamazepine
- Primidone
- Topiramate
- Modafinil
- Some antiretrovirals (e.g. ritonavir, nevirapine) – full details are obtainable from www.hiv-druginteractions.org
- St John's Wort — potency varies; CSM advises *non-use*

Broad-spectrum antibiotics (less important) that interact with COCs.
- Ampicillin, amoxycillin and related penicillins
- Tetracyclines
- Broad-spectrum cephalosporins

Note that none of the proton-pump inhibitors – including lansoprazole – are now regarded as having any clinically important enzyme induction effect. Moreover ethosuximide, valproate and clonazepam and most newer anti-epileptic drugs (including vigabatrin and lamotrigine) do not pose this problem. Among antimicrobials, co-trimoxazole, erythromycin and clarithromycin actually tend to raise blood levels of EE, although not dangerously (grapefruit juice is similar!). So all should preferably be taken at least 3 hours after pill taking.

Short-term use of any interacting drug/long-term broad-spectrum antibiotics

Extra contraceptive precautions are advised during treatment and should then be continued for a further 7 days, with elimination of the next PFI as appropriate from Figure 11, based on when in the pill packet the last potentially less effective pill was taken. The stakes are particularly high with **griseofulvin** because of its strong teratogenicity.

Rifampicin is such a powerful enzyme inducer that even if it is given only for 2 days (e.g. to eliminate carriage of meningococcus), increased COC elimination by the liver must be assumed for 4 weeks thereafter, i.e. as though it had been given long term (see below). The extra contraception (e.g. condoms) should be continued to cover all that time therefore, plus *also* elimination of any expected PFIs.

With **broad-spectrum antibiotics** the large-bowel flora responsible for recycling oestrogens are reconstituted with resistant organisms within about 2 weeks. In practice, therefore, if COCs are commenced in a woman who has been taking a tetracycline long term, there is no need to advise extra contraceptive precautions. There is a potential problem (now believed to involve very few women but clinically we never know which) in the reverse situation, i.e. when the tetracycline is first introduced to treat a long-term COC user. Even then, extra precautions need only be sustained for a maximum of 14 days plus the usual 7 days, with elimination of the next PFI if the 2 weeks of antibiotic use involved any of the last seven pills of a pack.

Long-term use of enzyme inducers

This applies chiefly to epileptic women and women being treated for tuberculosis. This is WHO 3, meaning that an alternative method of contraception is preferable and should always first be discussed: such as an IUD or the injectable, DMPA. With the latter there need be *no special advice* to shorten the injection interval, (see p. 83), even for patients needing **rifampicin** or **rifabutin,** whose effects on the COC are such that long-term users are strongly advised against it.

For the remainder, if the combined pill is nevertheless chosen, it is recommended to prescribe an increased dose, usually 50–60 µg oestrogen initially and also advise one of the tricycle regimens described above. This reduces the number of contraceptively risky PFIs, which is particularly appropriate for epileptic women since the frequency of attacks is often reduced by the maintenance of steady hormone levels. The PFI should also, logically, be shortened at the end of each tricycle. At the MPC we advise that the next packet should begin after 4 days, even if the withdrawal bleed has not stopped.

Only one 50 µg pill remains on the UK market (Table 3) and metabolic conversion of the prodrug mestranol to EE is only about 75% efficient. Therefore Norinyl-1 is almost identical to Norimin. So, one is usually forced to construct a 50 or 60 µg regimen from two sub-50 µg products, e.g. 2 × Microgynon 30 or a Femodene™ (Schering Health Care) plus a Femodette tablet (see Table 3). As this practice is unlicensed, this is named-patient use and the guidance on p. 141 should be followed.

BTB may occur; indeed, it could have been the first clue to a drug interaction. If the long-term user of an enzyme inducer develops persistent BTB, the first step is a speculum examination and all the other assessments in the checklist on p. 50. It may *very rarely* then be worth trying an even higher dose, combining pills to a total oestrogen content of 80 or 90 µg (a rare maximum). This is following the usual policy (pp. 47–8) of giving the minimum dose of both hormones to be just above the threshold for bleeding. The woman can be reassured that she is metaphorically 'climbing a down escalator' – her increased liver metabolism means that she should still in reality be receiving a low-dose regimen. **But**, there is some uncertainty here, the criteria of p. 141 must be rigidly applied, and surely a change of method would nearly always be preferable!

Discontinuation of enzyme inducers after long-term use

It has been shown that 4 or more weeks may elapse before excretory function in the liver reverts to normal. Hence, if any of these drugs has been used for 1–2 months (or at all in the case of a rifamycin), there should be a delay of about 4 weeks before returning to a standard low dose regimen. This period should be increased to 8 weeks after more prolonged use of enzyme inducers. In all cases there should be no PFI gap between the higher dose and low-dose packets [see (5) of Table 7, p. 46].

Special considerations

Duration of use

Many important benefits are enhanced as duration of COC use increases. There need be no restriction on duration of use for healthy non-smokers up to the maximum age (see below). Even for smokers or others with arterial risk factors, age seems a more important consideration than duration of use.

Maximum age for COC use

In selected healthy migraine-free, non-smokers, with modern pills and careful monitoring, the many gynaecological and other benefits of COCs are now felt to outweigh the small, though increasing, cardiovascular (and breast cancer) risk of a modern pill up to age 51, which is the mean age of the menopause. Depending on her choice, an appropriate COC (most commonly a 20 µg product such as Mercilon or Femodette, see p. 36) may thus be preferable (WHO 2) to hormone replacement therapy (HRT) up to the age of 51, for women who need contraception as well as a supplement to diminished ovarian function. Smokers above the age of 35 are a different matter. Pending more data, if they request a hormonal contraceptive they should use a progestogen-only method – an IUD or IUS might be even better (or perhaps the partner should have a vasectomy?).

Beyond 51 years of age, the age-related increased COC risks are usually unacceptable for all, since fertility is now so low that simple, virtually risk-free contraceptives will suffice, e.g. barriers or Delfen™ (Janssen-Cilag) foam (p. 138) – or the POP (p. 66).

Most forms of HRT are not contraceptive, but may be indicated combined with one such simple contraceptive if oestrogen is no longer being supplied by the COC. Of course, the IUS plus HRT combination (p. 113) is a winner here, since it safely supplies contraceptive HRT plus also, usually, highly acceptable oligo-amenorrhoeia. With such combinations it may never be necessary to know the precise time of final ovarian failure. The contraception component may simply be stopped either:

- after the latest age of potential fertility (58 years); **or**
- earlier, after waiting the 'officially approved' 1 year after the last bleed or any hormones.

Raised follicle-stimulating hormone (FSH) measurements, although more reliable above the age of 50–51, are never diagnostic. There are preliminary data to suggest that a raised FSH at the very end of the PFI may indicate that the ovaries have ceased to function. This should be confirmed by a repeat FSH 6 weeks off all therapy. Above 50 years of age, a second high FSH result along with vasomotor symptoms and amenorrhoea (to date and continuing) is *suggestive* of final ovarian failure. The woman should be warned that the *risk of later ovulation cannot be excluded*, but she may choose to discontinue contraception, or to use a simple contraceptive for a further 1 year.

Another protocol, which may be more acceptable to some, is at the age of 51 to switch from a COC to a POP. If amenorrhoea and vasomotor symptoms follow (either immediately, or months or years later), FSH measurements while still taking the POP can help to confirm ovarian failure (see p. 79).

Congenital abnormalities and fertility

Any possible effect of COCs on congenital abnormalities is hard to establish because it is so difficult to prove a negative, and 2% of all full-term fetuses have a significant malformation. Even with exposure during organogenesis, meta-analyses of the major studies fail to show an increased risk. If present it must be very small.

Used *prior to* the conception cycle, the conclusions of a WHO scientific group have not since been challenged – namely, that there is no good evidence for any adverse effects on the fetus of COCs. It can do no harm if a woman stops COCs for 2 or more months before conception, but there is no objective evidence that it is worth the effort: certainly, any woman who finds herself pregnant immediately after stopping COCs should be strongly reassured.

Fertile ovulation can be minimally delayed, yet there is no evidence that COCs can cause permanent loss of fertility. Indeed a large study, Farrow et al (2002) *Hum Reprod* **17**: 2754–61) showed that more than 5 years use of the COC before the 8497 *planned* conceptions was associated with a *decreased* risk of delay in conceiving, even for nulliparous women!

What about 'taking breaks' to optimize fertility?

If a woman feels more comfortable taking a routine break from the COC, we should always help her to find a satisfactory contraceptive alternative. However, there is no known benefit to fertility or indeed to health from taking short elective breaks of 6 months or so every few years, as was once recommended. In one study, a quarter of young women who took such breaks had unwanted conceptions. It helps some women to be reminded that regular PFIs give the body plenty of breaks from the COC anyway, totalling 130 every 10 years!

Screening

After the age of 20, cervical screening should be performed regularly, as recommended for all sexually active women. *Routine* breast or bimanual examinations in asymptomatic Pill-takers are uncalled for, the latter because the disorders causing detectable pelvic masses or tenderness are, as listed on p. 10, actually *less frequent* in COC-takers than in others.

Summary

The first visit for prescription of COCs is by far the most important and should never be rushed. Often it is useful to share it between the doctor and practice nurse. The newer long-term and 'forgettable' contraceptive choices should always be included in the discussion (see p. 4), despite the woman's presenting request for what she happens to know about (the Pill).

If the Pill remains her choice, along with discussing the risks and benefits, and fully assessing her medical and family history, all at her level of understanding, there is much ground to cover:

Take-home messages for a new pill-taker.
- Your FPA leaflet: this is not to be read and thrown away, it is something to keep safely in a drawer somewhere for ongoing reference
- The Pill only works if you take it correctly: if you do, each new pack will always start on the same day of the week
- Even if bleeding, like a 'period', occurs (BTB), carry on Pill taking – ring for advice if necessary. Nausea is another common early symptom. Both usually settle as your body gets used to the Pill
- Lovemaking during the 7 days after any packet is only safe if you do go on to the next one: otherwise (if you are stopping the Pill for any reason), start using condoms after the last pill in the pack
- Even if your 'period' (withdrawal bleed) has not stopped yet, never start your next packet late. This is because the PFI is obviously a time when your ovaries are not getting the contraceptive, so might anyway be beginning to escape from its actions.
- For what to do if any pill(s) are more than 24 hours late, see p. 57
- Other things that may stop the Pill from working include vomiting and some drugs (pp. 58, 60–4)
- See a doctor *at once* if the things an p. 53 occur
- As a one-off manoeuvre you can shorten one PFI to make sure all your future withdrawal bloods avoid weekends
- You can avoid bleeding on holidays etc by running packs together (discuss this with whoever provides your pills, if you want to continue missing out 'periods' long term, i.e. tricycling)
- Good though it is as a contraceptive, the Pill does not give adequate protection against Chlamydia and other STIs. Whenever in doubt, especially with a new partner, use a condom *as well*
- Finally, always feel free to telephone or come back at any time (maybe to the practice nurse) for any reasons of your own, including any symptoms you would like dealt with

---

Thereafter there are really only three key components to COC monitoring during follow-up:

- BP (pp. 42, 54);
- headaches (pp. 42–5);

- identification and management of any new risk factors/diseases/side effects.

In conclusion, no matter how carefully those with contraindications are excluded, a few women will experience adverse effects. Repeated presentation with multiple side effects may indicate the need for a different method. However, excessive anxiety and possible psychosexual aspects may need to be discussed.

OTHER COMBINED METHODS

Transdermal combined hormonal contraception

EVRA (Janssen-Cilag) is an innovative transdermal patch delivering EE with norelgestromin, the active metabolite of NGM. The daily skin dose of 150 µg norelgestromin and 20 µg EE produces blood levels in the range of those after a tablet of Cilest but without either diurnal fluctuations or the oral peak dose given to the liver. Pending more specific research information, all the absolute and relative contraindications and indeed most of the above practical management advice about the COC apply, with obvious minor adjustments, to this new product. It appears to be relatively oestrogen-dominant, with a bleeding and non-bleeding side-effect profile very like Cilest itself – plus about 2% of women in the trials had local skin reactions which led to discontinuation.

The patch has excellent adhesion even in hot climates and when bathing or showering; the incidence of detachment of patches was 1.8 % (complete) and 2.9 % (partial). In the pooled analysis of the RCT studies the Pearl index for consistent users of EVRA was similar to the oral pills – and less than 1 per 100 woman-years. Interestingly, in the clinical trials, one third of the few failures occurred in the 3% weighing above 90 kg. In my view this apparently reduced effectiveness contraindicates EVRA for such women who are at least WHO 3 for VTE risk at that level of BMI anyway.

Transvaginal combined hormonal contraception

Already available in some European countries and the USA, NuvaRing (Organon) is expected in the UK in 2004 or 2005. It is a combined vaginal ring which releases etonogestrel (3-keto-desogestrel) 120 µg and EE 15 µg per day, thus equating to some degree with 'vaginal Mercilon'. It is normally retained (though there is an option of removing it during sexual activity) for 3 weeks and then taken out for a withdrawal bleed during the fourth.

Pending more dedicated information, all the absolute and relative contraindications, and most of the above practical management advice about the COC, must be presumed to apply to NuvaRing. It appears to be relatively oestrogen dominant, with a side-effect profile very like Mercilon itself. In studies at the MPC and elsewhere it proved very popular, with excellent cycle control and once again a failure rate comparable to the COC.

Maintenance of efficacy of NuvaRing.
- Expulsions were a problem for some (usually parous) women, primarily during the emptying of bowels or bladder, and therefore readily recognized.
- As with the COC, it will still be essential never to lengthen the contraception-free (ring-free) interval. If for any reason this exceeds 8 days, I advise extra precautions for 7 days. EC should be added if there has been sexual exposure during any ring-free time of more than 8 days
- On the COC model (see Figure 11), provided a ring has been intravaginal for a full 7 days, after premature expulsion/removal – even for up to 5 days – contraceptive efficacy should be restorable just by immediate insertion of a new ring
- There would of course be the possibility of offering it in a tricycle way (as with the COC), meaning the consecutive use of three or four rings before the break
- Absorption problems, vomiting/diarrhoea and broad-spectrum antibiotics have no effect on this method's efficacy
- Additional contraception is still advised with simultaneous enzyme-inducer therapy

---

Intramuscular combined hormonal injectables

The pill by injection, known as Lunelle™ in the USA, is a monthly combined injectable giving monthly bleeds, using medroxyprogesterone acetate plus an oestrogen (oestradiol cypionate). Its arrival in the UK is likely to be delayed at least until a planned self-injector system is perfected.

There are six varieties of POP available (Table 8), five of the old type and the sixth, Cerazette, is new, a primarily anovulant product, very different and therefore mainly dealt with at the end of this section. Unless otherwise stated the abbreviation POP will refer to the old-type POPs.

Table 8
Available POPs.

Product	Constituents	Course of treatment
Noriday[TMa]	350 μg norethisterone	28 tablets
Micronor[TMb]	350 μg norethisterone	28 tablets
Femulen[TMa]	500 μg etynodiol diacetate	28 tablets
Neogest[TMc]	75 μg dl norgestrel*	35 tablets
Norgeston[TMc]	30 μg levonorgestrel	35 tablets
Cerazette[TMd]	75 μg desogestrel	28 tablets

*Equivalent to 37.5 μg LNG.
[a]Searle; [b]Janssen-Cilag; [c]Schering Health Care; [d]Organon.

Mechanism of action and the maintenance of effectiveness

The mechanism of action is complex because of variable interactions between the administered progestogen and the endogenous activity of the woman's ovary. Outside of lactation, fertile ovulation is prevented in at least 60% of cycles. In the remainder there is reliance mainly on progestogenic interference with mucus penetrability, backed by some anti-nidatory activity at the endometrium. The starting routines are summarized in Table 9.

If POPs are taken absolutely regularly each day within a time span of 27 hours, without breaks and regardless of bleeding patterns, they are almost as effective as COCs, especially for those aged 30 and over.

In the UK the Oxford/FPA study reported a failure rate of 3.1 per 100 woman-years between the ages 25 and 29, but this improved to 1.0 at 35–39 years of age and was as low as 0.3 for women over 40 years of age. Realistically, most users are probably not as meticulous as those married middle class women; therefore, since almost

Table 9
Starting routines for POPs.

Condition before start	Start when?	Extra precautions?
Menstruation	Day 1 of period	No
	Day 2 or later	7 days
	Any time in cycle ('Quick start')	7 days†
Postpartum*		
No lactation	Usually day 21	No
Lactation	Day 21 – maybe later if 100% lactation	No
After induced abortion/ miscarriage	Same day	No
After COCs	Instant switch	No
Amenorrhoea (e.g. postpartum)	Any time‡	7 days

*Bleeding irregularities minimized by starting at or after the 4th week.
†Can start any day in selected cases **if** the prescriber is satisfied there has been no conception risk up to the starting day.
‡If prescriber is confident that no blastocyst or sperm is already in upper genital tract. (See p. 46, final footnote to Table 7).

everyone has a mobile phone, I now routinely advise dedicating one alarm to 'POP-taking time'.

Studies are suggestive, but not conclusive, that the failure rate of old-type POPs may be higher with increasing *weight*, as was well established for progestogen rings and some implants. Pending more data, I now recommend the use of Cerazette for women over 70 kg (irrespective of height), especially if they are young. This is preferable to taking two POPs, but one POP suffices anyway during established breastfeeding or in older women, particularly above the age of 45.

Interference with contraceptive activity as a result of missed pills, vomiting or drug interaction is believed to start within as little as 3 hours but is corrected adequately, as far as the mucus is concerned, if renewed Pill taking is combined with extra precautions for just 48 hours. In 2003, the Faculty of FP and the UK FPA decided to follow WHO's Practice Recommendations (see WHO's website, p. 142). So after missing a POP for more than 48 hours the woman should:

- take that day's pill immediately and the next one on time;
- Use added precautions for the next 2 days.

If there has already been intercourse without added protection between the time of first potential loss of the mucus effect through to its restoration by 48 hours then:

- EC is also advised.

However, except for pill omissions beyond 24 hours, pending more data, in my opinion EC would be unnecessary in Cerazette-users (p. 79), or during full lactation with ordinary POPs.

According to the lactational amenorrhoea method (LAM),

even without the POP there is only about 2% conception risk if – and *only* if – all three LAM criteria continue to apply, namely:

- *amenorrhoea, since the lochia ceased;*
- *full lactation – the baby's nutrition effectively all from its mother;*
- *baby not yet 6 months old.*

This is why postcoital contraception would very rarely be indicated for missed POPs during full lactation. But because breastfeeding varies in its intensity, it is still usual if a tablet is 3 hours late to advise additional precautions during the next two tablet-taking days.

During lactation, with all POPs including Cerazette the dose to the infant is believed to be harmless, but this aspect must always be discussed. The least amount of administered progestogen gets into the breast milk if a LNG POP is used. The quantity is the equivalent of only one POP in 2 years, considerably less than the progesterone level found in formula feeds. If EC is required (rarely, see above) by a breastfeeding mother, she may wish for just 24 hours to express and discard her breast milk, though even then there is no evidence that this higher LNG dose would cause her baby any harm.

In young and highly fertile women using old-type POPs it is advisable to recommend switching back to the COC (or, perhaps, Cerazette) for greater effectiveness as soon as the infant starts to be weaned, ideally no later than the first bleeding episode.

Broad-spectrum antibiotics do not interfere with the effectiveness of POPs or indeed any progestogen-only method. Another highly effective contraceptive method would normally be advised during use of enzyme inducers such as *rifampicin* and *griseofulvin*. Long-term treatments with enzyme inducers is WHO 3, but if a suitable altern-ative is not found increasing the dose is an option: usually to two POPs, or perhaps two Cerazettes, daily, the choice depending on consideration of all relevant factors includ-ing lactation and the woman's body weight, age and likely fertility. See also, as usual, p. 141

Advantages and indications

The indications (WHO 1 or sometimes WHO 2) for POP or Cerazette use are as considered in the Box below.

Indications for POP or Cerazette use.
- Lactation, where the combination even with ordinary POPs is extra effective, indeed as good as the COC would be in non-breastfeeders
- Side effects with, or recognized contraindications to, the combined pill, in particular if oestrogen related. As EE-free products do not appear to significantly affect blood-clotting mechanisms it may be used by women with a definite past history of VTE and a whole range of disorders predisposing to arterial or venous disease (pp. 37–40, 44, 78). *Good counselling and record keeping are essential*
- Smokers above 35 years of age
- Hypertension, whether COC related or not, controlled on treatment
- Migraine, including focal aura varieties (the woman may continue to suffer migraines but the fear of an EE-promoted thrombotic stroke is eliminated)
- Diabetes mellitus (DM), but caution WHO 3 or 4 if significant DM of tissue damage (see Box below)
- Sickle cell disease
- Obesity, but then usually prescribing Cerazette (see text)
- At the woman's choice

Contraindications

Absolute contraindications are few and are given in the Box below.

Absolute contraindications for POP and Cerazette use.
- Past severe arterial diseases, or current very high risk thereof
- Any serious adverse effect of COCs not certainly related solely to the oestrogen (e.g. progestogen allergy, liver adenoma)

- Recent breast cancer not yet clearly in remission (see below)
- Acute porphyria, if history of actual attack (progestogens as well as oestrogens are believed capable of precipitating these), otherwise WHO 3 (see below)
- Recent trophoblastic disease until hCG is undetectable in blood as well as urine, but earlier use is acceptable in some countries, including the USA (see p. 17)
- Undiagnosed genital tract bleeding
- Actual or possible pregnancy
- Hypersensitivity to any component

In my view there are 5 strong relative contraindications (WHO 3)

Strong relative contraindications for POP and Cerazette use.
- Acute porphyria, latent, with no previous attack (and caution, forewarning/monitoring); POP is also usable in all the non-acute porphyrias
- Sex-steroid-dependent cancer, including breast cancer, in complete remission (WHO advises 5 years). In all cases, agreement of the relevant hospital consultant should be obtained and the woman's autonomy respected: record that she understands it is unknown whether progestogen alone alters the recurrence risk (either way)
- Enzyme inducers [two POPs can be taken (see above) but another method such as an IUD or IUS would be preferable]
- Past symptomatic functional ovarian cysts
- Previous treatment for ectopic pregnancy; *however*, this is an **indication** for Cerazette!

Although it is now well established that the risk of ectopic pregnancy is actually reduced among POP users, which is why the condition is not WHO 4, it can be reduced still further by methods which markedly reduce fertilization rates (such as the COC, DMPA, Cerazette or Implanon™). These allow better preservation of the precious remaining Fallopian tube, especially in nulliparae. The increased frequency of *symptomatic cysts* with POPs can lead to problems in the differential diagnosis from ectopic pregnancy. (Persistent cyst/follicles which are commonly detected on routine ultrasonography can be disregarded when they cause no symptoms.)

The remaining **relative** contraindications, in which the POP method is generally WHO 2 and may certainly be used with good supervision are as given in the Box below.

Mild relative contraindications for POP and Cerazette use.
- Past VTE or severe risk factors for VTE; in fact, I would argue that this is an Indication (see above)
- Risk factors for arterial disease; more than one risk factor can be present, in contrast to COCs
- Current liver disorder even if there is persistent biochemical change
- Most other chronic severe systemic diseases (but WHO 3 or even 4 if the condition causes significant malabsorption of sex steroids)

Follow-up and management of side effects

Apart from the complaint of *breast tenderness*, which is usually transient but may be recurrent and can sometimes be overcome by changing POPs, without doubt the main side effect is *menstrual irregularity*. With advance warning this may be tolerated. Improvement appears more likely with Cerazette, based on the RCT comparing it with a LNG POP; however, the difference was only evident when users persevered beyond 6 months. More than half of old-type POP users do have a cycle of between 25 and 35 days. A few women experience very prolonged or heavy bleeding, and if this is not relieved by changing the POP another method should be offered.

Except during full lactation, prolonged spells of *amenor-rhoea* occur most often in older women. Once pregnancy is excluded, the amenorrhoea must be the result of anovulation and so signifies very high efficacy. The method can be continued unless there are marked symptoms of hypo-oestrogenism (which is most uncommon, see below).

BP is checked initially, but if normal at 6 months does not need to be taken more than annually at most. When raised during COC use it usually reverts to normal on POPs. Indeed, if it does not the woman most probably has essential hypertension.

There are negligible changes to most *metabolic variables.* If *complete amenorrhoea* occurs, more commonly with Cerazette than other POPs, what happens to oestrogen levels? It appears that with all POPs (and Implanon), FSH is not completely suppressed even during amenorrhoea, leading to enough follicular activity at the ovary to maintain adequate mid-follicular phase oestrogen levels. Pending more data, there is not therefore the concern about arterial and bone health which is as yet unresolved for DMPA (see pp. 85–7).

Establishing ovarian failure at the menopause is less important than with the COC (p. 65), since all the POPs are safe enough products to continue using well into the late 50s. Hence, first switching to any POP from the COC (see p. 66) can be a reassuring way to manage that often difficult transition out of the reproductive years.

If later a non-contraceptive HRT method is desired, and there is amenorrhoea above the age of 50 on an old-type POP (not the pituitary-suppressing Cerazette), a high blood FSH measurement (more than 30 IU/l) suggests ovarian failure. Two high values 6 weeks apart, especially if there are vasomotor symptoms, would make the likelihood of a later ovulation very low. Should the FSH be found to be low, however, this suggests that some simple additional contraceptive should still be used, along with the planned HRT.

Cerazette

Mechanism of action and maintenance of effectiveness

This useful new product containing 75 μg desogestrel rewrites the text books about POPs, mainly because it blocks ovulation in 97% of cycles and had a Pearl index failure rate in the pre-marketing study of only 0.17 per 100 woman-years (in perfect users not also breastfeeding). This makes it somewhat like 'Implanon by mouth'; and it is indeed useful as a way of advance testing the acceptability of Implanon in selected cases, though only with respect to hormonal side effects (and with a risk of Cerazette-induced BTB).

At the time of writing, the CSM in the UK has not yet approved for Cerazette any lengthening beyond 3 hours in the time before a single delayed pill triggers the need for added precautions – though at least these are now only advised for 2 days with any variety of POP. While therefore encouraging potential users to be as meticulous as that with their Cerazette taking, a major advantage is its suitability for many young and highly fertile users for whom we would previously not even have suggested a POP. Realistically, despite tricks like setting one of their mobile phone alarms, busy or scatty individuals are sure to miss some POPs but they are much more likely to get away with it on Cerazette.

Return of fertility with all POPs including Cerazette is rapid. Indeed, from the contraceptive point of view, fertility after stopping must be assumed to be almost immediate.

Starting routines are unchanged from those in Table 9.

Advantages and indications

For a start, Cerazette must be free of all the risks attributable to EE, plus no effects on BP have been reported. Hence, it can be used in many cases where a COC is WHO 4 or 3 but a Pill method with greater efficacy than ordinary POPs is desired.

In particular, given the earlier discussion about POPs and body weight, Cerazette would now be my first choice for a woman weighing over 70 kg unless she was breastfeeding or over 45 years of age.

Cerazette also usually ablates the menstrual cycle like COCs but again without using EE, so it has potentially beneficial effects and can be tried (not always successfully) in a range of menstrual disorders, especially:

- dysmenorrhoea;
- menorrhagia;
- premenstrual syndrome (PMS).
- Cerazette may also be a good alternative primarily anovulant method when there is a past history of ectopic pregnancy or for maintenance therapy in endometriosis

Unwanted effects

As with all progestogen-only methods, irregular bleeding remains a very real problem. Indeed, this is the one area showing no great advantage in the pre-marketing comparative study with LNG 30 µg users. The drop-out rate for changes in bleeding pattern showed no difference, but there was a useful trend for the more annoying frequent and prolonged bleeding experiences to lessen with continued use, and at 1 year around 50% had either amenorrhoea or only one or two bleeds per 90 days.

Despite this higher incidence of (more acceptable) amenorrhoea than with existing POPs, Cerazette like other POPs and Implanon still appears to provide adequate follicular-phase levels of oestradiol, so there are at present no concerns with respect to osteoporosis.

Contraindications

These, whether WHO 4, 3 or 2 are very similar to those for old-type POPs. The main difference is that Cerazette is more effective, making it positively suitable for a past history of ectopic pregnancy and for young fertile women with complicated structural heart disease. However, functional ovarian cysts still occur in some Cerazette-users.

In summary, this may well become a first-line hormonal contraceptive for many women. However there is no indication in my view to use it rather than a cheaper old-type POP in lactation or in older women, especially in those above 45 years of age. One cannot expect to improve upon 100 percent contraception, which in combination with an ordinary POP these two states do (almost) provide!

Injectables

In the UK the only injectable currently licensed by the CSM for long-term use is DMPA, and it has been given additional approval as a first-line contraceptive. It has been repeatedly endorsed by the expert committees of prestigious bodies, such as the International Planned Parenthood Federation and WHO. DMPA is even safer than COCs, in spite of the adverse publicity it often receives.

Anxiety about this method was generated by animal research of very doubtful relevance to humans. WHO data indicate that DMPA-users have a *reduced risk of cancer*, with no overall increased risk of cancers of the breast, ovary or cervix, and a fivefold reduction in the risk of carcinoma of the endometrium (relative risk 0.2). There is still the possibility of a weak cofactor effect on breast cancer in young women similar to that with COCs (see pp. 11–15). However, this is unproven and the apparent association may be due to surveillance bias in early years of use by the younger women.

Administration, mechanism of action and effectiveness

There are two injectable agents available: DMPA 150 mg every 12 weeks, and Noristerat™ (Schering Health Care) (norethisterone enanthate) 200 mg every 8 weeks, both given by deep intramuscular injection in the first five days of the menstrual cycle. Injections may also be given beyond day 5 with 7 days added precautions if it is near certain that a conception risk has not been taken. The injection sites should not be massaged.

The effectiveness of DMPA is extremely high among reversible methods (0–1 failure per 100 woman-years), primarily because it functions by causing anovulation, backed by similar effects on the mucus and endometrium to the COC.

Potential drug interactions

Contrary to previous advice, since the liver ordinarily clears the blood reaching it completely of the drug – and enzyme inducers cannot increase clearance beyond 100% – there is no requirement to shorten the injection interval. This applies even to users of **rifampicin or rifabutin** (p. 63).

Timing of the first dose

I recommend timings as outlined in the Box below:

Timing of the first injectable.
- In *menstruating women* the first injection should normally be given before day 5 of the cycle; if given on day 5 or later advise 7 days extra precautions (see below for management of overdue injections)
- If a woman is on a *COC* or *POP* or *Cerazette*, the injection can normally be given any time, with no added precautions
- *Postpartum* (when the woman is *not* breastfeeding) or after a *second-trimester abortion*, the first injection should normally be at about day 21, and if later with added precautions for 7 days. If later and still amenorrhoeic, pregnancy risk must be excluded (p. 46, footnote). Earlier use is sometimes clinically justified
- *During lactation* the POP is preferable to DMPA; but – best given at 6 weeks – it is not inhibited and the dose to the infant is small and believed to be entirely harmless
- *After miscarriage* or a *first-trimester abortion*, 7 days extra precautions advice is not necessary unless the injection is given on day 7 or later

---

Overdue injections of DMPA with continuing sexual intercourse.

WHO in their Practice Recommendations are unconcerned by injections up to 2 weeks late. Due to conceptions reported as early as the end of the 13th week I remain unrepentant and still advise the simple protocol given in the Box below.

Protocol for late injection.
- From day 85 to 91 (13th week), injection **plus** condoms or equivalent to be used during the next 7 days
- From day 92 to 98 (14th week), injection if negative sensitive (25 mIU/l) pregnancy test **plus** emergency contraception by hormone or more rarely copper IUD as appropriate **plus** condoms for 7 days
- Beyond day 98, the next injection is best postponed until there has been a total of 14 days of safe contraception or abstinence since the last sexual exposure **plus** a sensitive pregnancy test is negative **plus** advising 7 days of added contraception e.g. with condoms (no EC would then be needed)

(see also p. 130).

In all circumstances, always counsel the women regarding possible failure and provide no guarantee that any fetus will be normal. Follow-up after a further two weeks or so, to exclude conception after all late injections, is a sensible precaution.

Advantages and Indications

DMPA has obvious contraceptive benefits (effective, 'forgettable'), but the data imply that it also shares most of the non-contraceptive benefits of the COC described on p. 10, including some protection against pelvic infection.

The main *indication* is the woman's desire for a highly effective method that is unaffected by enzyme inducers and independent of intercourse, when other options are contraindicated or disliked. Injectables may be used despite a past history of ectopic pregnancy or, like all other progestogen-only methods, of thrombosis (see earlier comments for the POP): they are ideal for many women who require effective contraception while waiting for major or leg surgery.

DMPA is positively beneficial in endometriosis, past symptomatic functional cysts, sickle cell anaemia and epilepsy, in which it often reduces the frequency of seizures.

Unwanted effects

The most significant are:

- irregular, sometimes prolonged bleeding;
- amenorrhoea and potential hypo-oestrogenism;
- weight gain (the latter can be marked in some cases).

Menstrual abnormalities remain the greatest obstacle to any large increase in the method's popularity. *Excessive bleeding* may resolve if the next injection is given early (but not less than 4 weeks since the last dose). At the MPC it is often found that giving additional oestrogen is more successful, either as EE 30 µg (as such or more usually within a pill formulation) or, if there is a past history of thrombosis or other WHO 4 contraindication to EE, as natural oestrogen (e.g. estradiol 50 µg by patch). Either is given daily for 21 days, after which there is a withdrawal bleed, usually for three cycles, and courses may be repeated if an acceptable bleeding pattern does not follow.

Amenorrhoea occurs in most long-term users and is usually very acceptable, with the explanation if necessary that 'menstruation has no excretory function or health benefits'.

There is a concern, however, that *prolonged hypo-oestro-*

genism through use of DMPA (with or without oligo-amen-orrhoea) might lead, by analogy with premature menopause, to some added risk of osteoporosis or, more importantly, arterial disease. There is no proof of this either way. A report by WHO in 1998 on heart disease in current users was somewhat reassuring, but more data are urgently needed. In the meantime, based on the precautionary principle, I recommend the protocol outlined in the Box below.

Protocol re potential oestrogen deficiency with DMPA

- First, consider if there are any potential WHO 4 contraindications: e.g. severe anorexia nervosa or steroid treatment above 5 mg daily, predisposing to osteoporosis; severe or multiple arterial disease risk factors. According to WHO, being over 45 years of age or (because of queries about achievement of peak bone mass) under 18 years of age is only WHO 2
- Otherwise, only after 5 years use should the issue normally be *reviewed* with the woman herself, or earlier if she has actual relevant symptoms (notably dryness of the vagina, hot flushes). The outcome of this discussion may be:
- the wish anyway to make a change to another method, which will of course restore oestrogen levels, either exogenously (e.g. COC) or from her own ovaries
- given the absence of any proof of any important risk and all the advantages of the method, some women will wish to continue, uncomplicatedly with DMPA alone, whatever the result of any test. If so, their view is simply noted carefully, with the plan only to raise the matter again if new data are published or after a further 5 years use
- in the (small) residual group only, if desired, the oestradiol level in a blood sample shortly before the next injection is measured. If the result is above 100 pmol/l and there are no symptoms, the woman may continue on DMPA and the test might be repeated routinely in about 5 years time. If the result is lower than 100 pmol/l the test is repeated. Two levels under 100 pmol/l are now taken as grounds for the still preferred course of a *change of method*; or, more controversially, if the woman insists, the use of add-back natural oestrogen HRT by any chosen route and usually continuously. Since it is *unlicensed* to use DMPA in this way, this must be on a named-patient basis (see p. 141)

Expensive *bone scans* or *blood lipid assays* are not indicated routinely, although they could be appropriate on *specific clinical grounds* (e.g. a bone scan for a thin teenage athlete or on the emergence of an anorexia history, lipids because of a new family history of heart attack).

Contraindications

Absolute contraindications for DMPA.
- Past *severe arterial diseases*, or *current very high risk* thereof (because of the evidence re low oestrogen levels coupled with reports of lowered HDL cholesterol)
- *Severe risk factor(s) for osteoporosis*, including *chronic steroid treatment* more than 5 mg per day
- Any *serious adverse effect of COCs not certainly related solely to the oestrogen* (e.g. progestogen allergy, liver adenoma)
- *Recent breast cancer* not yet clearly in remission (see below)
- *Acute porphyria, with or without history of actual attack* (progestogens as well as oestrogens are believed capable of precipitating these)
- *Recent trophoblastic disease* until hCG is undetectable in blood as well as urine, but earlier use is acceptable in some countries, including the USA (see p. 17)
- *Undiagnosed genital tract bleeding*
- Actual or possible *pregnancy*
- *Hypersensitivity* to any component

Relative contraindications for DMPA.
- According to degree, *arterial disease risk* is WHO 3 or 2 (except as above)
- Short-term *steroid treatment, recovered anorexia nervosa, athletes with amenorrhoea* are all usually WHO 3; *under 18 or over 45 years of age* are WHO 2 with respect to the bones (see above). Indeed, over 45 years of age is arguably WHO 3, given the increasing arterial disease risk
- *Active liver disease* with abnormal liver function tests – caution required (WHO 3 or 2)
- DMPA is usable in all *non-acute porphyrias* (WHO 2) but unlike POPs should **not** be used in *latent acute porphyria* (WHO 4)
- *Sex-steroid-dependent cancer*, including breast cancer, in complete remission is WHO 3 (WHO advises 5 years); however, a POP is preferable (lower dose, more reversible, see p. 77)

- *Unacceptability of menstrual irregularities*, especially cultural/religious taboos associated with bleeding, or *amenorrhoea*
- *Obesity*, although further weight gain is not inevitable
- Past *severe endogenous depression*
- *Planning a pregnancy in the near future*

Counselling

Three particular points must always be made to prospective users:

- *The effects, whether wanted (contraceptive) or unwanted, are not reversible* for the duration of the injection: this fact is unique among current contraceptives
- After the last dose *conception is commonly delayed with a median delay of 9 months*, which is of course only 6 months after cessation of the method, but in some individuals it could be *well over 1 year*. A comparative study in Thailand showed that almost 95% of previously fertile users had conceived by 28 months after their last injection, therefore refuting allegations of permanent infertility caused by the drug
- Weight gain is probable due to increased appetite, so it is ideal (and can really work) to plan pre-emptively to start taking **extra** exercise!

Follow-up

Aside from ensuring the injections take place at the correct intervals (if not see p. 84), follow-up is primarily advisory and supportive. Excessive bleeding and amenorrhoea are managed as already described. BP is normally checked initially but there is absolutely no need for it to be taken before each dose as studies fail to show any hypertensive effect. An annual check is reasonable as well-woman care.

Contraceptive implants

The implant route remains very useful, despite the allegations made in recent years by the media and some lawyers.

Implants contain a progestogen in a slow-release carrier, made either of dimethylsiloxane (as in Norplant™ (Hoechst Marion Roussel) with six implants, and the very similar two-rod Norplant II™, now called Jadelle™) or ethylene vinyl acetate (EVA; Implanon). Inserted into the medial upper arm, after an initial phase of several weeks giving higher blood levels, they deliver almost constant low daily levels of the hormone (Figure 14).

Mechanism of action and effectiveness

Implanon is the only marketed implant in the UK. It works primarily by ovulation inhibition, supplemented by the usual mucus and endometrial effects. It is a single 40 mm rod, just 2 mm in diameter, inserted subdermally straight from a dedicated sterile pre-loaded applicator with a cleverly shaped wide-bore needle (Figure 14), by a simple injection/withdrawal technique. The implant contains 68 mg of etonogestrel – the new name for 3-keto-desogestrel – and so has much in common with Cerazette. This is dispersed in an EVA matrix and covered by a 0.06 mm rate-limiting EVA membrane.

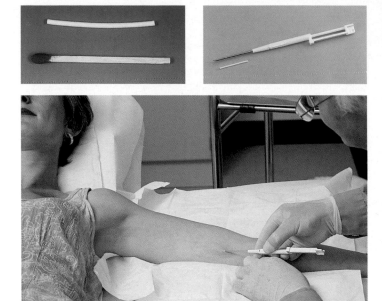

Figure 14
Implanon (by courtesy of Organon Laboratories Ltd).

Effectiveness of Implanon.
- The duration of use is for 3 years, with the unique distinction of a zero failure rate in the pre-marketing trials, though the 95% confidence interval ranges up to 7 in 10 000. Nearly all 'failures' subsequently reported were pregnant already or failures to insert
- In international studies, serum levels tended to be lower in heavier women, but there were no failures, whatever the BMI! I advise consideration of earlier replacement (after 2 years) in young fertile women weighing over 100 kg **if** they start cycling regularly in the third year
- If enzyme-inducer drug treatment is necessary, additional contraceptive precautions are recommended. One option is to prescribe an added daily Cerazette tablet (unlicensed use, see p. 141)

Though the implant is much easier than Norplant to insert or remove, specific training is essential and cannot be obtained from any book. In a comparative study, the mean insertion time was 1.1 minutes and the mean removal time 2.6 minutes (range 0.2–20.00 minutes).

Removal problems correlate with initially too-deep insertion. Beware particularly of (indeed, consider referral for) the thin or very muscular woman with very little subcutaneous tissue. Insertion can easily permit a segment of the rod to enter the (biceps) muscle with deep migration following.

Timing of Implanon insertion
Insertion of Implanon is usually in the UK timed as below:

Timing of Implanon insertion.
- *In the woman's natural cycle*, day 1–5 is usual; if day 5 or any day later (assuming no sexual exposure up to that day) I recommend additional contraception for 7 days. Natural-cycle insertions are a logistic and conception risk nightmare! (see next bullet)
- If a woman is *on COC or Cerazette*, the implant can normally be inserted any time, with no added precautions. Since Cerazette is much like 'Implanon by mouth', it has added value here compared to old-type POPs: it can usefully be tried for 1–2 months after Implanon counselling, to evaluate **non-bleeding** side effects – as well as providing interim contraception. But see p. 80.
- *Following delivery or second-trimester abortion* (not breastfeeding) insertion on about day 21 is recommended, and if later with additional contraception for 7 days. If later and still amenorrhoeic, pregnancy risk should be excluded (p. 46, final footnote)
- If *breastfeeding* insert after 6 weeks. The manufacturer urges caution: uncertainty about the (probably nil) effects of the tiny amount of etonogestrel reaching the breast milk must be discussed (as for the POP, which would be no less effective)
- Following *first-trimester abortion*, immediate insertion is best, or up to 7 days; on day 7 or later an added method such as condoms is recommended for 7 days.

Advantages and indications

The main *indication* is the woman's desire for a highly effective method without the finality of sterilization that is independent of intercourse, when other options are contra-indicated or disliked .

> **Indications for Implanon.**
> - Above all it provides efficacy and convenience: if the bleeding pattern suits it is a 'forgettable' contraceptive
> - Long action with one treatment (3 years), high continuation rates
> - Absence of the initial peak dose given orally to the liver
> - Blood levels are steady rather than fluctuating (as with the POP) or initially too high (as injectables); this minimizes metabolic changes
> - Oestrogen-free, therefore usable if history of VTE (this is only WHO 2, in my opinion)
> - Median systolic and diastolic BP were unchanged in trials for up to 4 years
> - Being an anovulant, special indications include past ectopic pregnancy and all the menstrual disorders which Cerazette (pp. 80–1) may also benefit. A preliminary trial with Cerazette can sometimes be useful (p. 80)
> - The implant is rapidly reversible: after removal serum etonogestrel levels were undetectable within 1 week. From the contraceptive point of view, return of fertility must be assumed to be almost immediate

Contraindications

> **Absolute contraindications (WHO 4) for Implanon.**
> - Any *serious adverse effect of COCs not certainly related solely to the oestrogen* (e.g. progestogen allergy, liver adenoma)
> - *Recent breast cancer* not yet clearly in remission (see below)
> - *Acute porphyria,* with history of actual attack
> - *Recent trophoblastic disease* until hCG is undetectable in blood as well as urine (but see p. 17)
> - *Known or suspected pregnancy*
> - Undiagnosed genital tract bleeding
> - *Hypersensitivity* to any component

The manufacturer adds '*severe hepatic disease*', which I classify as WHO 2 (see below) or at most WHO 3, and '*active venous thromboembolic disorder*', which in my view should also be WHO 2. There is no evidence that Implanon would increase VTE risk.

Relative contraindications are as for Cerazette (pp. 77–8), since, like it but unlike DMPA, Implanon is immediately reversible.

Relative contraindications (WHO 3) for Implanon.
- *Acute porphyria, latent,* with no previous attack (and caution, forewarning/monitoring); Implanon is also usable in all the non-acute porphyrias
- *Sex-steroid-dependent cancer, including breast cancer,* in complete remission for 2 years (WHO advises 5 years). In all cases agreement of the relevant hospital consultant should be obtained and the woman's autonomy respected: record that she understands it is unknown whether progestogen alone in Implanon alters the recurrence risk (either way)
- *Enzyme inducers* [an extra daily Cerazette can be taken (see above), but another method such as an IUD or IUS would be preferable]
- Past *symptomatic* functional ovarian cysts – might recur on Implanon implantation, especially in the third year

Relative contraindications (WHO 2) for Implanon.
- *Past VTE or severe risk factors for VTE*; in fact, I would argue that this is an Indication, see above
- *Risk factors for arterial disease*; more than one risk factor can be present
- *Current liver disorder* even with persistent biochemical change
- Most other *chronic severe systemic diseases*
- *Unacceptability of irregular menstrual bleeding* remains a problem with all progestogen-only methods, certainly including Implanon

Follow-up and management of side effects

Counselling should explain the likely changes to the bleeding pattern and the possibility of 'hormonal' side effects (see below). This discussion should as always be backed by a good leaflet, such as the FPA one, and well-documented.

No treatment-specific follow-up is necessary (including no need for BP checks). However, there should be an explicit open-house policy so the woman knows she can return at any time to discuss possible side effects, without any provider pressure to persevere if the woman really wants the implant removed (the standard for the maximum wait for which should be no more than 2 weeks).

In the pre-marketing RCT of Implanon with Norplant the *bleeding patterns* were very similar, with one main difference. As expected for an anovulant method, amenorrhoea was significantly more common (20.8 versus 4.4%). The infrequent bleeding and spotting rate was 26.1%. Normal cycling was reported by 35% of women, but the combined rates for the more annoying 'frequent bleeding and spotting' and 'prolonged bleeding and spotting' totalled 18% with Implanon. The best short-term treatment is cyclical COC therapy, logically with two to three cycles of Mercilon, after which the bleeding may (or sometimes may not!) become acceptable.

Minor side effects reported in frequency order were: acne, headache, abdominal pain, breast pain, 'dizziness', mood changes (depression, emotional lability), libido decrease, hair loss. In a comparative study the mean *body weight increase* over 2 years was 2.6% with Implanon and 2.9% with Norplant, but in a parallel study, users of an IUD showed weight increases of 2.4%. Though this implies a normal increase over time, by 24 months 35% had put on more than 3 kg. Weight seems to be less of a problem than with DMPA, though some individuals do find their weight gain unacceptable.

Since Implanon suppresses ovulation and does not supply any oestrogen, the same questions as with DMPA arise over *possible hypo-oestrogenism* (p. 86). However, it appears that, like Cerazette and other POPs, the suppression of FSH levels is not complete, allowing sufficient follicular oestrogen: and the findings on both oestrogen levels and bone density are very reassuring:

Local adverse effects, such as infection of the site, migration, difficult removal and scarring are very infrequent. Discomfort at insertion and removal can be minimized by good training.

Intrauterine contraception

Copper-bearing devices

'Time to forgive the intrauterine device (IUD)'. This headline to a recent article says it all. Actually, there are 150 million users worldwide, but the lion's share is in just one country, China. Is the difference between less than 1% of sexually active users in USA but 20% in France explicable by some important difference between the French and the US uterus? Hardly! The US Dalkon Shield catastrophe explains much. But in many countries women in their 30s have not been requesting IUDs because they were told in their 20s to avoid that method. However, a woman in her later reproductive years with, say, two or three children is the ideal user, the devices have changed somewhat but she has too

Advantages of copper IUDs.
- Safe: mortality 1:500 000
- Effective:
  immediately
  postcoitally (unlike the LNG IUS)
  highly, with T-Safe Cu 380A, cumulative failures at 7 years only 1.4/100 women
- No link with coitus
- No tablets to remember
- Continuation rates high and duration of use can exceed 10 years
- Reversible, even when removed for one of the recognized complications

(commonly she also has less exposure to pelvic infection risk). Some doctors are complying too readily with requests for male or female sterilization which originate partly out of myths about the intrauterine alternative. Leaving aside the significant advance represented by the LNG IUS, too few women know that the latest **banded** *copper* IUDs are, in practice, more and not less effective than the COC and truly comparable to reversible sterilization.

Choice of devices and effectiveness

In the UK, the 'gold standard' among copper IUDs for a parous woman with no menstrual problems is the *banded* T-Safe Cu 380A (Figure 15). Of statistically similar efficacy to the LNG IUS, this is much more effective (Figure 16) than the *old* Nova T in preventing both intrauterine and (dangerous) ectopic pregnancies. The Nova T 380, with a greater surface area of copper wire is its replacement. In the only RCT comparing Nova T 380 with T-Safe

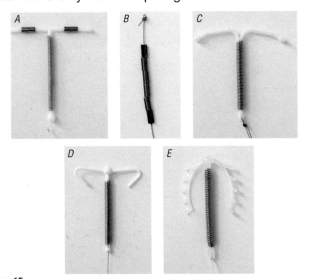

Figure 15
The T-Safe Cu 380A (A) and GyneFix (B), (banded) The Nova-T380 (C), Flexi-T 300 (D) and Multiload 375 (E) (unbanded). (Reproduced with kind permission of Elsevier and thanks to FP Sales, Oxford for supply of the devices.)

Pregnancies and ectopics

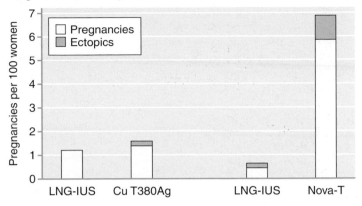

Figure 16
Five-year cumulative gross intrauterine and ectopic pregnancy rates per 100 women: for 1124 women using the LNG IUS versus 1121 using the Cu T 380Ag (a clone of T-Safe Cu 380A) on the left; and another 1821 women with the LNG IUS versus 937 using the old Nova T on the right. [Data from two RCTs (Sivin et al 1990. Contraception 42: 361–78. Andersson et al 1994. Contraception 49: 56–72.)]

Cu 380A (unhelpful names!), the wired IUD had a failure rate (3.6 per 100 women to 3 years) more than twice that of the banded one, a significant difference.

In Sivin's study (Figure 16) the cumulative failure rate of the T-Safe Cu 380Ag to 10 years was only 1.4 per 100 women (compare a mean rate of 1.8 per 100 women at 10 years after female sterilization in the CREST study, *American J of Obs & Gynaecology* 1996; **174**: 1161–70). There were no failures at all after year 5! And the fact that it has been UK-licensed for 8 years, and definitely usable at least to 10 years, constitutes a very real advantage, since:

> insertion and reinsertion procedures have been shown capable of causing almost every known IUD side effect.

GyneFix (also banded and about to be licensed for 10 years), shares that advantage (p. 109).

The Multiloads, even the 375 thicker wire version, were also significantly less effective than the T-Safe Cu 380A in WHO studies, with no evidence of the expected better expulsion rate. Flexi-T 300 is cheap and easy to fit, so suitable for short-term use as an emergency contraceptive, but is *not banded* and has a reportedly high expulsion rate.

Mechanism of action

Appropriate studies indicate that copper IUDs operate primarily by preventing fertilization. Their effectiveness when put in postcoitally indicates that they can also act to block implantation. However, this seems to be a rare back-up mechanism when devices are *in situ* long term.

As in any given cycle this IUD might be working through the block of implantation, there is a small risk of iatrogenic conception if a device is removed after mid-cycle. Ideally, therefore, women should use another method additionally from 7 days before planned device removal, or removal should be postponed until the next menses. If a device must be removed earlier, hormonal postcoital contraception may be indicated.

Influence of age

Copper IUDs, like all contraceptive methods, are more effective in the older woman because of declining fertility. Over the age of 30 there is also a reduction in rates of expulsion and of PID, which is not believed to be the result of the older uterus resisting infection but because the older woman is generally less exposed to risk of infection (whether through her own lifestyle or that of her only partner).

Unwanted effects of copper IUDs

The main medical problems are listed in the Box below. This is a remarkably short list as compared with hormonal methods.

> **Main problems with copper IUDs.**
> 1. *Intrauterine pregnancy*, hence miscarriage risks
> 2. *Extrauterine pregnancy*, though likelihood actually *reduced* in population terms
> 3. *Expulsion*, hence the risks of pregnancy/miscarriage
> 4. *Perforation*
>   risks of pregnancy
>   risks to bowel/bladder
> 5. *Pelvic infection* – though as with (2), IUD is not causative
> 6. *Malpositioning* [which predisposes to (1), (3) and (7)]
> 7. *Pain*
> 8. *Bleeding*
>   increased amount
>   increased duration

Note: all of the first six problems have the risk (directly or indirectly) of *impairing future fertility*. Moreover, they must be excluded as diagnoses before pain and bleeding are ascribed to side effects of this method.

In situ conception

If the woman wishes to go on to full-term pregnancy, after a pelvic ultrasound scan the device should normally be removed. This is counterintuitive, because one would think it would increase the miscarriage rate. In fact, the data for all devices studied show that the miscarriage rate is at least halved by removal of the device in the first trimester. For example, with the Copper T 200 device the normal rate of spontaneous abortion is 55%, dropping to 20% if the device was removed. The woman should of course be warned that an increased risk of miscarriage still remains.

If the woman is going to have a termination of her pregnancy, her IUD (or IUS) can be removed at the planned surgery; but it is safest to remove it before any medical abortion. If the threads are already missing when she is seen and other causes are excluded, aided by an ultrasound scan (see below), the pregnancy is at increased risk of second-trimester abortion (which could be infected), and antepartum haemorrhage and premature labour.

If the woman goes on to full term it is essential to identify the device in the products of conception. If it is not found, a postpartum X-ray should be arranged in case the device is embedded/malpositioned or has perforated. There have been medicolegal cases when this was not done, leading either to problems from an undiagnosed perforation or to unnecessary tests and treatments for 'infertility' when only one IUD was removed for a wanted pregnancy (leaving a much earlier malpositioned device *in situ*).

There is no evidence of associated teratogenicity with conception during or immediately after use of copper devices, or indeed of cancer developing in the uterus of long-term users.

IUDs with 'lost threads'
Often the threads are, in fact, present, although perhaps short or drawn up into the canal. If not, this symptom of 'lost threads' links together points (1), (3) and (4) in the Box on p. 99. There are at least six causes of this condition, three with and three without pregnancy (see Box below, p. 101). An intra-abdominal IUD is just as useless at stopping pregnancy as one that has been totally expelled. More commonly the woman is already pregnant and the threads have been drawn up or the device has altered its position *in situ*. So the slogan is:

> The woman with 'lost threads' is either already pregnant or at risk of becoming pregnant

Once pregnancy has been excluded the management is summarized in Figure 17. First, insert a long-handled Spencer–Wells forceps into the cervical canal and open the jaws carefully under direct vision. The threads were

'Lost threads' — six possible causes.

Pregnant
Unrecognized expulsion + pregnancy
Perforation + pregnancy
Device *in situ* + pregnancy

Not pregnant
Unrecognized expulsion + not yet pregnant
Perforation + not yet pregnant
Device *in situ* + malpositioned or threads short (in uterus, if not found in cervical canal)

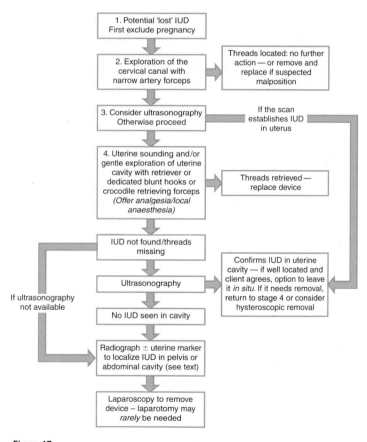

Figure 17
Management of 'lost' IUD threads.

found this way in about 40% of the women referred to the specialized 'lost threads' clinic at the MPC, meaning that they need never have been referred. In most of the remainder the thread was drawn down and the device removed – the Emmett design of thread retriever remains available. Appropriate analgesia is important: as a routine we give mefenamic acid 500 mg about 30 minutes before the examination but, in addition, local anaesthesia should be *offered* (see below).

If these manoeuvres fail, referral to the hospital gynaecologist may be necessary. In a study at the MPC only 2.5% of 350 *in situ* IUDs required general anaesthesia for removal, and a similarly low rate should be the norm. Investigations that may be helpful include ultrasound scan and an X-ray (another IUD may sometimes usefully be inserted as a uterine marker).

Perforation has a general estimated risk whether for framed or frameless devices of about 1 per 1000 insertions, but the exact rate depends crucially on the skill of the clinician. Perforated devices should now almost always be removable at laparoscopy.

PID
This is the great fear we all have about IUDs. Just as the Pill has been blamed for problems we now know were due to smoking, copper IUDs have been blamed for infections that were really acquired sexually (see the Chinese evidence, discussed below).

Much of the anxiety derived from the Dalkon Shield disaster, but this was a unique device with a polyfilamentous thread, increasing the risk of transfer of potential pathogens from the lower to the upper genital tract. Modern copper devices have a monofilamentous thread. They provide no protection against PID (in contrast to the LNG IUS – see below) and the infections that occur may perhaps be more severe as a result of the foreign-body effect, yet they do not themselves cause infection.

In a classic WHO study, Farley et al [(1992) *Lancet* **339**: 785–8] reported on a database from WHO RCTs, including approximately 23 000 insertions worldwide, and in every country the same pattern emerged (Figure 18). There was an IUD-associated increased risk of infection for 20 days after the insertion. However, the weekly infection rate 3 weeks after insertion went back to the same weekly rate as existed before insertion, i.e. the norm for that particular society. In China there were no infections diagnosed at all in spite of 4301 insertions. In another two contemporary studies from China a further 3300 IUD-users were followed for over a year, with again no cases of PID.

These findings are interpreted as follows: the post-insertion infection 'hump' cannot be the result of bad insertion technique, restricted to doctors outside China. Much more likely, although the doctors in all the centres were searching for

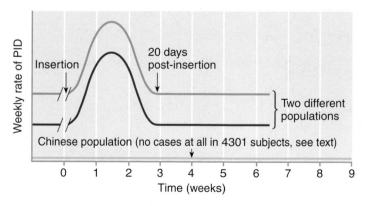

Figure 18
WHO study of 22 908 IUD insertions (4301 in China) in Europe, Africa, Asia and the Americas. PID, pelvic inflammatory disease. Note the weekly rate of PID returns to the preinsertion background rate for the population studied.

truly monogamous couples, they were only successful in this search in China (during the 1980s when China was practically an STI-free zone – China is no longer unique in this respect today). In the other countries, PID-causing organisms (especially *Chlamydia trachomatis*) are presumed to have been present in a proportion of the women. The process of insertion would interfere with natural defensive mechanisms (as has been confirmed when there is instrumentation in other contexts, such as therapeutic abortion). This would enable organisms to spread from the lower genital tract, where they had previously resided asymptomatically, into the upper genital tract, so causing the PID.

WHO findings of PID and IUDs.
- IUDs cannot, intrinsically, be the cause of PID: otherwise how could there have been so many as 7600 Chinese users in the 1980s and not a single attack?!
- The greatest risk is in the first 20 days, most probably caused by pre-existing carriage of sexually transmitted infections
- Risk thereafter, as with pre-insertion, relates to the background risk of STIs (high in Africa, but so low in mainland China in the 1980s that it seems to have been absent in the study population)

Therefore, the evidence-based policy should be that:

- Elective IUD insertions and **reinsertions** should always occur through a 'Chinese cervix', i.e. one that has been established to be pathogen-free, so hopefully eliminating the post-insertion 'hump' of infection in Figure 18

In practice, practical implications are as given in the Box below.

Practical implications of IUD insertion.
- Prospective IUD users should *always* be verbally screened, meaning a *good sexual history.*
- 'When did you last have sex with someone different?' (meaning more if within the past 3 months); **also**, and this is the thorny one we all tend to leave out:
- 'Do you ever wonder if your partner has or will have another sexual

---

relationship?' (Reworded as appropriate, and always with the utmost tact)

- In high prevalence populations (say greater than 5% incidence – and it is around twice that in most recent UK surveys of the under 25s) this should *often* be backed by modern DNA-based (LCR or PCR) screening, at least for *Chlamydia trachomatis*, before both IUD insertions and **reinsertions**
- Recent exposure history or evidence of a purulent discharge from the cervix indicates referral for more detailed investigation at a genitourinary medicine (GUM) clinic
- If *Chlamydia* is detected the woman should be investigated for linked pathogens at a GUM service, necessary treatment and contact tracing arranged, and the IUD insertion postponed. In emergency contraception cases (p. 126) screen but treat anyway before the result is available (e.g. with azithromycin 1 g stat)
- The cervix should be cleansed very thoroughly (primarily physically, by swabbing) before the device is inserted, with minimum trauma following the manufacturer's instructions
- In addition to the routine 6-week follow-up visit, a first post-insertion visit should logically be arranged at 1-2 weeks, designed to identify any women with post-insertion infection (during the 'hump' of Figure 18). As a minimum, the woman should be given clear details of the relevant symptoms of PID, and instructed as routine to telephone the practice nurse about 1 week post-insertion

The *Chlamydia* screen can of course be omitted if, for example, the woman is over 40 years of age and the sexual history of 'symmetrical' monogamy is strong, and especially if her family is considered complete.

It is surely suboptimal to fit IUDs or IUSs without *Chlamydia* pre-screening being the norm. The added expenses of the test and any antibiotics are readily offset by the bargain cost of the T-Safe Cu 380A: about £1 per year over 10 years. 'Blind' prescription of an appropriate antibiotic is necessary in emergency cases, but the screening should still be done. Otherwise contact tracing is impossible and reinfection will simply occur later, the woman becoming one of the regular weekly cases after 'the hump' (Figure 18).

Actinomyces-*like organisms (ALOs)*

These are sometimes reported in cervical smears, more commonly with increasing duration of use of either IUDs or IUSs. If reported, the protocol in the Box below is recommended.

First part of protocol on detection of ALOs.
- Call the woman for an extra consultation and *examination, particularly bimanually*
- If there are relevant symptoms or signs (pain, dyspareunia, excessive discharge, tenderness, any suggestion of an adnexal mass) then an ultrasound scan should be arranged, with a low threshold for gynaecological referral. After preliminary discussion with the microbiologist, the device should be removed and sent for culture. Treatment will have to be vigorous, usually prolonged, if pelvic actinomycosis is actually confirmed – it is a potentially life-threatening and fertility–destroying condition, although very rare

---

More usually, the ALO finding occurs in asymptomatic and physical sign-free women – who stay that way. Over-reaction might cause more morbidity, through pregnancy, than through actinomycosis. In a study reported from the MPC in 1984 three groups of women were followed up: one group was simply monitored (and the ALO finding commonly persisted) and in the other two groups the device was removed with or without immediate reinsertion of another copper IUD. No antibiotics were given. In both latter groups (and in larger studies of simple IUD removal) follow-up smears were free of ALOs.

Second part of protocol on detection of ALOs.
When there are no positive clinical findings, in consultation with the woman decide between **EITHER:**
- Simple removal with or without reinsertion, and without antibiotic treatment
- Advise the woman, along with written reference material, about the relevant symptoms which should make her *seek a doctor urgently* and tell them that she recently had an IUD or IUS plus ALOs
- Repeat a cervical smear after 3 months (it will nearly always be

---

negative) with a re-check bimanual examination. Both smear-taking and IUD follow-up then revert to normal intervals.

OR

- Leave the IUD or IUS alone after the initial thorough and fully reassuring examination, if in any doubt backed by ultrasound
- Advise the woman, along with written material, about the relevant symptoms which should make her *seek a doctor urgently* and tell them that she has been followed up with an IUD or IUS plus ALOs
- Arrange meticulous 6-monthly follow-up, including a check for symptoms and bimanual examination every time
- While the original IUD/IUS remains *in situ*, cervical smears are bound to continue showing the ALOs; so they are repeated at normal screening intervals.

In either case keep a good quality record of the consultation.

Ectopic pregnancy

Is this problem caused by copper IUDs? This is another myth. The main cause is previous tubal infection with one or both tubes being damaged. The non-causative association with IUDs comes about because they are even more effective at preventing pregnancy in the uterus than in the tube.

Ectopic pregnancies are actually reduced in number because very few sperm get through the copper-containing uterine fluids to reach an egg, so very few implantations can occur in any damaged tube. However, there are even fewer implantations in the uterus. Thus, in the ratio of ectopic to intrauterine pregnancies, the denominator is even lower than the numerator, allowing the ratio to increase, even though both types of pregnancy are actually reduced in frequency. The estimated rate of ectopic pregnancy for sexually active Swedish women seeking pregnancy is 1.2–1.6 per 100 woman-years. The risk in users of either the T-Safe Cu 380A and its clones or of the

LNG IUS is estimated as 0.02 per 100 woman-years, which is at least 60 times lower.

Clinically, caution about ectopic pregnancy is still necessary.

Any IUD-user with pain and a late period or irregular bleeding has an ectopic pregnancy until proved otherwise. (A past history is a WHO 3 relative contraindication to the method since there are even better anovulant options, particularly in nulliparae).

Pain and bleeding

Pain and bleeding in IUD-users signify a dangerous condition until proved otherwise

As well as excluding conditions such as infection and an ectopic pregnancy or miscarriage, consider malpositioning of any framed device (contrast GyneFix, see below) which can cause pain through uterine spasms.

Copper devices do increase the duration of bleeding by a mean of 1–2 days, and they also increase the measured volume of bleeding by about one third. In a population of copper-IUD-users, haemogloblin levels tend to fall, and those with losses above 80 ml/cycle are prone to frank anaemia. Bleeding problems usually settle with time. If they do not it may be necessary to change the method of contraception, perhaps to the LNG IUS method (see below). Drug treatments may reduce the loss but are not very satisfactory long term. The most successful therapies are mefenamic acid 500 mg 8 hourly and tranexamic acid 1–1.5 g 8 hourly.

Duration of use

Studies regularly show reduced rates of discontinuation with increasing duration of use, whether for expulsion, infection or pain and bleeding or indeed pregnancy. Coupled with the fact that most IUD complications are insertion related, it is good news that the banded devices T-Safe Cu 380A and GyneFix may both be used for 10 years or longer (see below).

Above the age of 40, the agreed policy, since a 1990 statement in *The Lancet* by the FPA and the predecessor body of the Faculty of FP and Reproductive Health Care, is:

> Any copper device (even a copper-wire-only type) that has been fitted above the age of 40 may be that woman's last device, which need never be changed, even though it is not licensed for that long (see p. 141)

(For duration of use of the LNG IUS in various situations (normally 5 years), see below.

GyneFix

This unique frameless device (Figure 19) features a knot that is embedded by its special inserter system in the fundal myometrium. Below the knot, its polypropylene thread bears six copper bands and locates them within the uterine cavity. It appears to retain the efficacy and other advantages of the T-Safe Cu 380A. But if properly implanted (by 'experts') there is the potential of a lower expulsion rate (as low as 0.4 per 100 woman-years in the first year of use) and there are no removals for pain of mechanical origin. Malpositioning is also less likely than with framed IUDs.

Special training for the implantation is essential, even by doctors fully experienced in inserting existing framed devices. The patient should be forewarned about easily unrecognized expulsion: being able to feel the threads is particularly important with this product.

Among over 250 users beyond 5 years in two studies, one in China and the other WHO-linked, only one conception occurred to 10 years. Hence, I am informed by the inventor

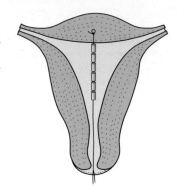

of GyneFix (Wildemeersch, personal communication 2003) that an application is in process for a 10-year licence.

The indications for GyneFix rather than T-Safe Cu 380A are considered below.

The levonorgestrel-releasing intrauterine system [LNG IUS, or Mirena™ (Schering Health Care)]

The LNG IUS is shown in Figure 20.

Method of action and effectiveness

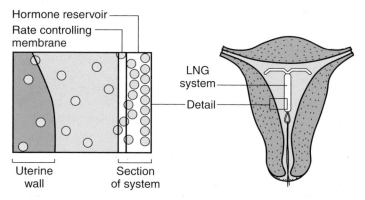

Hormone reservoir

Rate controlling membrane

Uterine wall

Section of system

LNG system

Detail

Figure 20
The LNG-releasing IUS (Mirena).

Advantages and Indications

The *contraceptive* advantages given in the above Box are, of course, shared with the T-Safe Cu 380A, which is the current gold standard for copper IUDs. However, this is where the similarity ends. It fundamentally 'rewrites the textbooks' about IUDs, really only sharing the intrauterine location and deserving a separate category (hence 'IUS').

The user of this method can expect the following advantages:

- *A dramatic reduction in amount and*, after the first few months (discussed below), *duration of blood loss.*
- *Dysmenorrhoea* is improved in most women and (for unexplained reasons) the *PMS* in some. The LNG IUS is the contraceptive method of choice for most women with *menorrhagia* or who are prone to iron-deficiency anaemia. It should be the first-line long-term primary care treatment for excessively heavy menses without major cavity distortion, for which it is now fully licensed in all circumstances

- *HRT:* by providing progestogenic protection of the uterus during oestrogen replacement by any chosen route it uniquely, before final ovarian failure, offers 'forgettable, contraceptive, no-period and no PMS-type HRT'. Although not yet licensed for the latter in the UK it may be used on a named-patient basis (p. 141), but never left *in situ* for longer than 5 years (see below)
- *Epilepsy:* in a small series at the MPC this was a very successful method for this condition, even in women on enzyme-inducer treatment (see Box on p. 111)
- It is, in short, a highly convenient and '*forgettable*' contraceptive (p. 4), – *with added gynaecological value.*

What about infection/ectopic pregnancy/risk to future fertility?

Although existing IUDs do not themselves cause PID, they fail to prevent it and there is a suspicion they sometimes worsen the attacks that occur. The LNG IUS may actually reduce the frequency of clinical PID, particularly in the youngest age groups who are most at risk. The risk is certainly not eliminated and condom use should still be advocated, but the data available make it possible to offer the LNG IUS to some young women requesting a 'forgettable' contraceptive who would not be good candidates for conventional copper IUDs. ALOs may be reported; a finding which should be managed as described on pp. 106–7.

The Progestasert and an experimental WHO device that released only 2 µg per day of LNG were both associated with an *increased* risk of extrauterine pregnancies. Copper-wire IUDs are an improvement, but the data published for this device show (like the banded copper IUDs) a *massive reduction* in that risk, which can be attributed to its greater efficacy by mechanisms that reduce the risk of pregnancy in any site, whether uterine or extrauterine. However, with a past history of an ectopic pregnancy, an anovulant method would be even better.

Unwanted effects of the LNG IUS

As with any intrauterine device, *expulsion* can occur and

there is the usual small risk of *perforation*, minimized by its 'withdrawal' as opposed to 'plunger' technique of insertion.

A more important problem is the high incidence in the first post insertion months of *uterine bleeding* which, although small in quantity, may be very frequent or continuous and can cause considerable inconvenience. In later months, amenorrhoea is commonly reported. For both of these effects, particularly the former, forewarned is forearmed, implying the need for good counselling. In my experience, women can accept the early weeks, even of very frequent light bleeding, as a worthwhile price to pay for all the other advantages of the method, provided they are well informed in advance of LNG IUS fitting, and coached and encouraged as appropriate while it is occurring. The amenorrhoea can be explained and interpreted to a woman as an advantage – gently debunking the myth that menstruation serves an excretory function – not an adverse side effect but a positive benefit of the method.

Women should also be forewarned that although this method is mainly local in its action it is not exclusively so. Therefore there is a small incidence of *'hormonal' side effects* such as bloatedness, acne and depression. These do usually improve, often within 2 months, in parallel with the known decline in the higher initial LNG blood levels. Some clinicians find that early removals for this particular reason can be minimized by each woman having a short preliminary trial with a LNG-containing POP.

Functional ovarian cysts are also more common, although they are usually asymptomatic. If pain results they should be investigated/monitored but will usually resolve spontaneously.

Contraindications
Many of the contraindications of this method are shared with copper IUDs. The additional few that are unique to

LNG IUS, due to the actions of its LNG hormone, are discussed in the Box below.

Absolute unique contraindications (WHO 4) for LNG IUS.
- Current *liver tumour* or *severe active hepatocellular disease* (the latter is arguably more usually WHO 3 in my view)
- Current *severe active arterial disease* (most cases would be WHO 3 not 4 in my view)
- Current *breast cancer* (LNG IUS usable on WHO 3 basis after 2 years remission in my view, but 5 years according to WHO)
- *Trophoblastic disease (any)* – WHO 4 while blood hCG levels are very high, as for other hormonal methods (UK advice), **but** no problem after full recovery
- *Hypersensitivity* to levonorgestrel

In addition, *the LNG IUS should not be used as a postcoital intrauterine contraceptive* (at least one failure has been reported); effective though it is in long-term use, it appears not to act as quickly as intrauterine copper does.

Relative contraindications for copper IUDs also apply to the LNG IUS method, but are usually less strong, except for bleeding and pain which are positive indications (WHO 1).

Duration of use of the LNG IUS in the older woman

The product is licensed for 5 years.

Use of the LNG IUS in the older woman (duration).
1. For contraception, use is evidence-based (see p. 111) but unlicensed for up to 7 years. Therefore the older woman fitted above the age of 40 might continue at least till then at her fully empowered request, but always on a named-patient basis (p. 141)
2. As part of HRT, current practice for safe endometrial protection would be always to change at 5 years
3. But if the LNG IUS is not being and will not be used for either (1) or (2), it could be left *in situ* for as long as it works, in the control of heavy and/or painful uterine bleeding, and then removed after ovarian failure can be finally assured (say at age 58)

Conclusions

This method fulfils many of the standard criteria for an ideal contraceptive (see Box on p. 115). It approaches 100% reversibility, effectiveness and even, after some delay, convenience. This is because, after the initial months of frequent uterine bleedings and spotting, the usual outcomes of either intermittent light menses or amenorrhoea are very acceptable to most women. Adverse side effects are few and, in general, they are in the nuisance category rather than hazardous.

Since the advent of the LNG IUS my own lecture entitled 'Contraception for older women and those with intercurrent diseases' has been considerably simplified.

However, this method does fail on some criteria, especially the fifth bullet point in the Box below. There is no known protection against sexually transmitted viruses (and no *complete* protection against other STIs). So the 'Double-Dutch' approach (see p. 6) remains relevant. We also eagerly await an implantable version (see legend to Figure 19).

The ideal contraceptive.
- 100% (self-) reversible
- 100% effective (with the default state as contraception)
- 100% convenient (forgettable, non-coitally related)
- 100% free of adverse side effects (neither risk nor nuisance)
- 100% protective against STIs
- Has other non-contraceptive benefits
- Maintenance free (needing no initial or ongoing medical intervention)

Which device?

The **T-Safe Cu 380A** really is the gold standard and should almost always be tried first if there are no reported menstrual problems – including postcoitally if the device is likely to be used long term. **Flexi-T 300** is the cheapest slim and extra-easy-to-fit option for *short-term* emergency contraception, though the **Nova-T 380** could also be used in that way.

If there **are** menstrual problems – meaning that in the woman's own view her periods are **either** too heavy **or** painful **or** both – then there is no contest, the **Mirena LNG IUS** should be chosen (see below). Another special indication can be to obtain contraceptive HRT before final ovarian failure.

In my view, **GyneFix** (by referral to a Level 2 service if necessary) is preferred in the cases described in the Box below.

Cases when the GyneFix device is preferred.
- Small uterine cavity sounding less than 6 cm
- Distorted cavity on an ultrasound scan (if an IUD is useable at all)
- Previous expulsion of any framed device (with implantation by an expert!)
- Previous history of removal of a framed device within hours or days of insertion due to excessive cramping
- Significant spasmodic dysmenorrhoea history, since at least the pain cannot be added to by any frame – **if** the LNG IUS is not acceptable – but the latter can be brilliant for menstrual **pain** with *or* without menorrhagia

---

Which user?

Main established contraindications to IUDs
Note the differences in comparison with the LNG IUS (below and on p. 114)

Absolute – but perhaps temporary – contraindications (WHO 4) for IUDs.
- Suspicion of pregnancy
- Undiagnosed *irregular genital tract bleeding*
- *Significant infection:* post-septic abortion, current pelvic infection or STI, undiagnosed pelvic tenderness/deep dyspareunia or purulent cervical discharge
- *Significant immunosuppression*, i.e. more profound than use of low-dose corticosteroids
- *Malignant trophoblastic disease*, with uterine wall involvement

Absolute permanent contraindications (WHO 4) for IUDs.
- *Markedly distorted uterine cavity*, or *cavity sounding to less than 5.5 cm* depth. (But only WHO 2 for GyneFIX)
- Known *true allergy* to a constituent
- *Wilson's disease* (copper devices only)
- Past attack of *bacterial endocarditis* or *after prosthetic valve replacement*

Relative contraindications (WHO 2 unless otherwise stated) for IUDs (a copper IUD is usable with caution).

1. *Nulliparity and young age, especially less than 20 years.* Though this is WHO 2 for fear of infection and the more serious implications with no babies yet, this just means 'Broadly usable'. Both IUDs and IUSs are used successfully by many (carefully selected) women

2. *Lifestyle of self or partner(s) risking STIs.* Combined with (1) this equates to WHO 4, rarely 3 (with committed condom use)

3. *Past history of definite pelvic infection*

4. Recent exposure to *high risk of a sexually transmitted disease* (e.g. after rape – WHO 3). In emergency situations, such as for postcoital contraception, copper IUD may be permissible (WHO 3) with full antibiotic cover (after microbiological swabs are taken)

5. *Known HIV infection.* While controlled by drug therapy this is only WHO 2. LNG IUS is better still because of reduced blood loss (added condom use routinely advised)

6. Past history of *ectopic pregnancy or other history suggesting high ectopic risk in a multipara* (WHO 3). T-Safe Cu 380A, GyneFix or LNG IUS are preferred IUDs; but it is even better to use an anovulant contraceptive, especially if nulliparous.

7. *Suspected subfertility already.* WHO 2 for any cause, or WHO 3 if it relates to a tubal cause

8. *Structural heart disease* with risk but no endocarditis history. WHO 3, but WHO 2 for LNG IUS. Full antibiotic cover for insertion as advised in the BNF, for IUS as well as IUD

9. *Any prosthesis which can be prejudiced by blood-borne infection*, e.g. hip replacement. IUDs are certainly usable, but termed WHO 2 to flag up preference for antibiotic cover for the insertion

10. *Between 48 hours and 4 weeks postpartum* (excess risk of perforation; WHO 3)

11. *Benign trophoblastic disease.* WHO 3 while blood hCG levels very high with possible weakening of the uterine wall, and WHO 4 for the LNG IUS: **but** no problem after full recovery

12. *Severe cervical stenosis* (WHO 3). Pretreatment with oestrogen may help

13. *Fibroids or congenital abnormality* with some but not marked distortion of the uterine cavity (see above). WHO 2 for framed IUDs or IUSs, WHO 1 for GyneFix

14. *Severely scarred/distorted uterus*, e.g. after myomectomy (WHO 3)

15. *Primary dysmenorrhoea.* GyneFix (which should not worsen this) or the LNG IUS (which may well be of benefit, provided the frame does not cause spasmodic pain)

16. *After endometrial ablation/resection* – risk of IUD becoming stuck in shrunken and scarred cavity. LNG IUS or GyneFix usable in selected cases

17. *Heavy periods, with or without anaemia* before insertion for any

reason, including anticoagulation. This is an *indication* for the LNG IUS (WHO 1)

18. *Endometriosis.* May be benefited by LNG IUS (WHO 1)
19. *Diabetes.* WHO 2 for infection risk, but the IUD and LNG IUS can be excellent choices
20. *Penicillamine treatment* for Wilson's disease (WHO 4 for copper IUDs anyway) or rheumatoid arthritis. 'Small print', unproven risk of causing copper IUD failure; LNG IUS not affected
21. *Previous perforation of uterus* This is WHO 2, almost WHO 1, at least for the small defect in the uterine fundus after a previous IUD perforation. Healing is so complete, it is usually difficult even to ascertain the precise site of the previous event.

Note: if copper IUD desired, GyneFix being frameless would often be preferable for numbers (13)–(16). The LNG-IUS is often best for (15)–(20).

Counselling, insertion and follow-up

Timing of insertions

- In the *normal cycle, timing* must avoid any potentially implanted pregnancy (p. 125) but otherwise it is a *myth* that insertion is best during menses (higher expulsion rates are reported, in fact). With copper IUDs (because they are such efficient postcoital methods) insertion can be at any time up to 5 days after ovulation, but not so with Mirena (see below)
- Postpartum insertions of IUD or IUSs are usually at 6 weeks (beware increased risk of perforation)
- Insertions can also be very successful (but only after preliminary counselling) at the time of termination of pregnancy if the uterus is clearly empty (ideally checked by on-the-spot ultrasound)

Insertion timing for the LNG IUS (Mirena): this should be no later than day 7 of the normal cycle, since it does not operate as an effective anovulant or postcoital contraceptive **and** because, in addition, any fetus might be harmed by conception in the first cycle (very high local LNG concentration). Later insertion is advisable only if there has been believable abstinence, with continued contraception (e.g. condoms) thereafter, for at least 7 days.

Helpful tip: ensure that *as a routine* all who plan to have this

LNG IUS are (started on) a more effective method than condoms, e.g. the combined pill or perhaps Cerazette, so insertion can be performed any time, without any logistic timing problems and conception anxiety.

Counselling and follow-up

After considering the contraindications, there should be an unhurried discussion with the woman of all the main points above, particularly regarding her infection risk and the importance of reporting pain as a symptom.

She should always be given a user-friendly back-up leaflet and assured that in the event of relevant symptoms or if she can (no longer) feel her threads she will always receive prompt advice, and, as indicated, a pelvic examination.

The only important routine *follow-up visit(s)* are early on, maybe at 1 week (though that is more usually a telephone contact, see p. 105), otherwise usually at 6 weeks after insertion. This is to:

- discuss with the woman any menstrual (or other) symptoms;
- check for (partial) expulsion;
- exclude infection, i.e. no relevant symptoms, tenderness or mass.

According to WHO there need be no planned visits thereafter, only the above open-house policy. This is fine for copper IUDs but extra visits in early months can be helpful for LNG IUS-users to maintain their motivation before any bleeding problems settle (see below).

Insertion of devices

A pocketbook such as this is not the right medium for teaching insertion techniques. The Faculty of FP training leading to the Letter of Competence in Intrauterine Contraception Techniques is strongly recommended. This is a one-to-one apprenticeship, supplemented by videos and preliminary practice with an appropriate pelvic model, following the illustrations for each product that are in the packet.

Training should now include more attention than in the past to the issue of analgesia; at the MPC women routinely receive mefenamic acid 500 mg while in the waiting room. Local anaesthesia by intracervical injection should be taught and offered as a choice. It should almost always be used if the cervix has to be dilated or the uterine cavity explored. Moreover, in my experience, women have always much preferred having the holding forceps applied to the site at 12 o'clock on the cervix *with*, rather than without, an initial 2 ml dose of 1% lignocaine.

Lignocaine jelly 2% [Instillagel™ (Clinimed)] inserted by quill seemed to help in a study from Leeds, but my experience suggests there may have been a Type-1 error, i.e. statistical significance by chance. It just does not seem to be as effective as a cervical block and also raises questions about upward transfer of organisms from the cervix.

Points relating chiefly to the LNG IUS
If the uterus feels bulky/irregular on bimanual examination (suggesting fibroids) arrange an ultrasound scan requesting description of the endometrial cavity. If it is distorted, refer, perhaps for GyneFix if menorrhagia is not reported. Also refer older women above the age of 40 with any irregular (not just heavy) bleeding for a preliminary hysteroscopy.

There is now an excellent one-handed inserter gadget for Mirena. The insertion tube is fairly wide (4.8 mm), meaning that a set of Hegar size 3–6 dilators should always be available and that the skills for effective local anaesthesia may be required especially in older nulliparae.

Once learned, all these specific skills – including the management of 'lost threads' – must be maintained by regular practice. As we have already noted:

Insertion can be a factor in the causation of almost every category of IUD problems – another reason to prefer long-lived devices!

Summary of intrauterine devices (IUDs) and systems (IUS.)

• Last 9 days of the cycle	Time of one of the main actions (**Beware!** It might be operating in any IUD-removal cycle)
• Main counselling point	Fertility (risk and importance thereof)
• Pregnancy, expulsion and infection	All less common with increasing age
• Most IUD problems	Insertion related
• Continuing *in situ* pregnancy	Gently remove IUD in first trimester
• Pain + irregular bleeding	Ectopic pregnancy or another serious cause?
• 'Lost threads'	Pregnant or at risk until proved otherwise
• Duration of use	Long-term use is best*, i.e. leave well alone, especially to avoid the risks of each new insertion

*Except with respect to ALOs (p. 106); also the LNG load of the Mirena LNG IUS cannot support a duration beyond about 7 years (see pp. 111, 114)

Postcoital contraception

The use of large doses of oestrogen is outmoded because of severe nausea and vomiting. Apart from mifepristone, a 'hot potato' politically so still unavailable for this use, three methods have now been shown to be effective: the insertion of a copper IUD, the combined oral emergency contraceptive (COEC) and the LNG-containing **progestogen-only emergency contraceptive (POEC)** (see Table 10). Marketed as Levonelle (2)™, both on prescription and in pharmacies, POEC has made COEC of interest only where the former cannot be 'constructed' by using multiple POP tablets.

The recent Faculty Guidance Document (2003) (FGD 2003) is invaluable to supplement this chapter and readily downloadable from www.ffprhc.org.uk.

An important finding for both hormone methods is that every 12 hours delay in treatment increases the failure rate by 50%. For providers, this means giving the first dose always as soon as possible, taking us back somewhat to the concept of the morning-after pill. But EC remains a better lay term, since it leaves open the facts that useful benefit can be obtained long after 24 hours (Table 11) and that there is an important copper IUD alternative which is not a pill at all.

Progestogen-only emergency contraception (POEC) – one hormone is best!

Effectiveness and unwanted effects

In the 1998 RCT by WHO, comparing around 1000 women given this method (POEC) and the same number given COEC after a single exposure, the dosage regimens and main findings were as in Tables 10 and 11. This study has now been amplified by a larger RCT totalling 4136 women in 10 countries, with randomization to mifepristone and *either* to LNG 1.5 mg stat or the more usual POEC – which is the same total dose in divided doses of 0.75 mg taken 12 hours apart [WHO (2002) von Hertzen et al. *Lancet* 2002; **360**: 1803–10]. There was absolutely no difference in efficacy (nor in side effects) detectable between the two regimens.

I would agree with FGD 2003 that this means that whenever compliance may be poor the single-dose regimen may be used. Moreover at the time of writing it is expected that the SPC will change shortly to make this the norm anyway.

The main advantages of POEC are reduced rates of the main side effects of nausea and vomiting. It is also more effective (99.6% when treatment began within 24 hours, compared with 98% for COEC – in the single-exposure circumstances of the 1998 WHO trial) and there are virtually, in ordinary practice, no contraindications to it.

If the woman is taking an *enzyme-inducer drug* (including St John's Wort), the doses with the hormonal methods should be increased by 50% (i.e. two tablets of POEC stat and one in 12 hours). No increase in dose is needed when non-enzyme-inducing *antibiotics* are in use.

Warfarin-users should have their INR checked in 3–4 days after POEC, since it may alter significantly.

Table 10

Choice of methods for postcoital contraception.

	POEC (Levonelle 2) LNG 0.75 mg ×2 12 hours apart	COEC (used only if POEC not available) Use Microgynon 30 or equivalent × 8 tablets in divided doses 12 hours apart	Copper IUD Immediate insertion
Normal timing after intercourse	Up to 72 hours but also usable up to 120 hours (see below)	Up to 72 hours	Up to 5 days, or 5 days after earliest calculated day of ovulation (see p. 125)
Efficacy (overall) within 72 hours	98.5–99%	97%	About 99.9%
Side effects	Nausea 23% (15%)* Vomiting 6% (1.4%)*	Nausea 51% Vomiting 19%	Pain, bleeding, risk of infection
Contraindications	• Pregnancy • Proven *severe* acute allergy to a constituent • Active acute porphyria with past attack • Active severe liver disease [More often, less severe degrees of the last 3 conditions are WHO 3 not 4]	• Pregnancy • Proven severe acute allergy to a constituent • Active acute porphyria • Active severe liver disease • Current focal migraine • Current sickle cell crisis	• Pregnancy • As for copper IUDs generally

WHO, (1998) *Lancet* 1998; **352**: 428–33.
*WHO (2002) *Lancet* 2002; **360**: 1803–10.
LNG = levonorgestrel; EE = ethinylestradiol.

Table 11

Relative efficacies in each 24-hour period (from WHO 1998).

Coitus to treatment interval	POEC (Levonelle 2)		COEC (Schering PC4)
	Failure rate among all-comers (%)	% of expected pregnancies prevented	Failure rate among all-comers
<24 hours	0.4	95	2
25–48 hours	1.2	85	4.1
49–72 hours	2.7	58	4.7
0–72 hours	1.1	80	
72–120 hours	2.4*	Not calculated (small nos, see text)	

Note: on the basis of previous research into conception probabilities, 92 out of each 100 presenting in the 1998 study would not have conceived after the single exposure if untreated. 'Expected pregnancies' therefore are the remaining 8%, as the denominator.
*WHO (2002) study.

Contraindications (see Table 10)

Absolute contraindications (WHO 4) to the hormone methods are almost non-existent; those that may just be are listed in Table 10. There is no upper age limit to any of the methods if sufficient risk of conception is present.

Current breast cancer and *trophoblastic disease with high hCG levels* are both WHO 3, given the immediate risks of pregnancy. In *breastfeeding* (see LAM, p. 75) conception risk is of course lowered: but if treatment is indicated the infant could be bottle-fed for 24 hours, with expression of the breast milk.

Copper intrauterine devices (IUDs)

Insertion of a copper IUD – not the LNG IUS (see p. 114) – before implantation is extremely effective. This means insertion *in good faith* up to 5 days after:

- the *first* sexual exposure (regardless of cycle length); **or**
- the (earliest) calculated ovulation day (i.e. soonest likely *next* menstrual start day, subtract 14 days and add 5).

It prevents conception in about 99.9% of women who present, or 98% of those who might be expected otherwise to conceive (compare with the right columns of Table 11) – even in cases of multiple exposure ever since the last menstrual period. The judge's summing up in a 1991 Court Case (Regina vs Dhingra) gives legal support to this policy:

> I further hold ... that a pregnancy cannot come into existence until the fertilized ovum has become implanted in the womb, and that that stage is not reached until, at the earliest, the 20th day of a normal 28 day cycle ...

Contraindications

The copper IUD method has recognized contraindications (pp. 116–18) and the risks of pain, bleeding or infection. So this option, though it should be offered, is not often chosen by nulliparous women. However, in selected individuals IUD insertion may be appropriate (in categories listed in the Box below). This should generally be after cervical swabs (at least for *Chlamydia trachomatis*) and in high risk cases – as many of these are – with prophylactic antibiotic cover (p. 105), and contact tracing if STI test results later prove positive.

Insertion, which might be difficult in a nullipara, can usually be arranged nearby at a convenient Level 2 service. This could even be some days later than presentation, given the ability to use IUDs later in the cycle, after ovulation (see above) – on day 16, say, in a woman with a 26-day shortest cycle, presenting say on day 14 after the sexual exposure on day 11. FGD 2003 recommends giving POEC as well in such cases, on the presentation day, as a holding manoeuvre.

Indications for EC by copper IUD.

- When maximum efficacy is the woman's priority – at her choice. FGD 2003 says it should be offered to all, even when presenting within 72 hours
- When exposure occurred more than 72 hours earlier, or in cases of multiple exposure since the LMP: Insertion may be up to 5 days after the earliest UPSI or, if there have been many UPSI acts, no later than five days after ovulation
- In many women, often not always parous, to be retained as their long-term method (although it may be right in many young women to remove it after their next menses, once they are established on a new method such as the COC or injectable). *Always try to insert a banded IUD where long-term use is a possibility* (see discussion pp. 96–7)
- Presence of absolute contraindications to the hormonal method (a very rare indication with POEC)
- After vomiting of either dose within 2 hours, in a case with particularly high pregnancy risk – repeating a dose after domperidone 10 mg (see below) might otherwise suffice

Summary: counselling and management

First, evaluate the possibility of sexual assault or rape. Then, in a context which preserves **confidentiality** – and feels that way to the client – using (crucially) a good leaflet, such as that of the FPA, as the basis for discussion, help the woman to make a fully informed and autonomous choice of EC method.

- Careful assessment of *menstrual/coital history* is essential. Probe for other exposures to risk earlier than the one presented with. Note: ovulation is such a variable event that most women are best treated whenever they present in the 'normal' cycle, in *marked contrast to the Pill cycle*, (see below).
- *Contraindications* (see Table 10 and associated text above): The *mode of action* may itself pose an absolute contraindication to some individuals. Most modern ethicists (and the present author) and the Law consider that blocking of implantation is contraception and not abortion. Moreover, in a given cycle, if the treatment is given definitely pre-ovulation, even though postcoitally, POEC's powerful prefertilization effects on ovulation and the cervical mucus can remove that concern.
- *Medical risks* should be discussed, especially:
  - *the failure rate* (see Table 11), but remind the woman that these figures relate to a single exposure – the failure rate is very close to nil for the IUD method;
  - *teratogenicity:* this is believed to be negligible – although there is no proof – because before implantation the hormones will not reach the blastocyst in sufficient concentration to cause any adverse effect. Follow-up of women who have kept their pregnancies has so far not shown any increased risk of major abnormalities above the background rate of 2%;
  - *ectopic pregnancy:* if this occurs it results from a pre-existing damaged tube and would almost certainly have happened anyway, with or without this (pre-implantation) treatment. However:

a past history of ectopic pregnancy or pelvic infection remains a reason for forewarning with any of the methods, even though WHO categorises this as WHO 1; and

all women should be warned to report back urgently if they get pain – and providers must 'think ectopic' whenever POEC fails or there is an odd bleeding pattern post-treatment;

- Even if the POEC method is used, advice should be given regarding *nausea and vomiting* (the former occurred in the WHO 2002 trial in about 15% of cases, vomiting in only 1.4 %). If an anti-emetic is requested, the best seems to be domperidone [Motilium™ (Sanofi Winthrop)], 10 mg with each dose. If either contraceptive dose is vomited within 2 hours, the woman may be given further tablets or, in a particularly high-risk case, a copper IUD should be inserted.

- *Contraception*, both in the current cycle (in case the POEC method merely postpones ovulation), often condoms, and *long-term* should be discussed. The IUD option covers both aspects. Inform that regular use of all approved methods by the end of a year will beat using EC every month. If the COC or injectable are chosen it should normally be started as soon as the woman is convinced her next period is normal, usually on the first or second day, without the need for additional contraception thereafter. But 'Quick start' is also an option (p. 46) in selected cases, on the named-patient basis (p. 141), with appropriate documented warnings.

The above highlights the importance of a good rapport, to obtain an honest and accurate coital/menstrual history and to promote effective arrangements for more effective future contraception.

- Women receiving POEC should be instructed to return if their expected period is more than 7 days late, or lighter than usual, or if they experience *pain.*

IUD-acceptors return usually in 4–6 weeks for a routine check-up and sometimes removal (see above).

Vaginal examination is very rarely necessary if the IUD method is not in the frame, and there are very good reasons to omit it, for example, in an anxious teenager. It should be done only if indicated in the individual case on gynaecological grounds.

Special indications
These apply to coital exposure when the following have occurred:

- **Omission of two or more COC tablets** after the PFI (see p. 54), or of two or more pills in the *the first 7 in the packet* (see Figure 11 p. 57 and associated text). After the emergency regimen the woman may return to her COC taking the appropriate day's tablet within 12 hours of the second POEC dose – subject to a 100% undertaking to return for follow-up 4 weeks later and also to use added precautions for the next 7 days. WHO states that up to four mid-packet pill omissions after seven tablets already have been taken never indicate emergency treatment, or even condoms. If 5 or more pills are missed during days 8 to 14, WHO considers that both POEC and 7 days of condom use may be appropriate. Towards the end of a packet, (days 15–21) simple omission of the next PFI will suffice (no matter how many pills have been missed, up to seven anyway!).
- **Delay in taking a POP tablet for more than 3 hours**, implying loss of mucus effect, followed by sexual exposure during the 48 hours before contraception is expected to be restored. Again, the POP is to be restarted immediately after the emergency regimen, 2 days added precautions are advised, and follow-up agreed. If the POP-user is fully breastfeeding (pp. 74, 75) these actions would only be contemplated if the POP is taken more than one day late (i.e. as for the COC).

- **Removal or expulsion of an IUD** before the time of implantation, if another IUD cannot be inserted for some reason.
- **Further exposure in the same cycle**, e.g. due to failure of barrier contraception after an emergency hormonal method has been given. Additional courses of POEC, for example, are supported by FGD 2003 'if clinically indicated' (and after every reasonable precaution to avoid treating after any possible implantation). But such additional use increased the failure rate to at least 0.8% per cycle in one study quoted by the Faculty of FP, and is once again outside the terms of the licence (see p. 141).
- **Use of POEC later than 72 hours after exposure.** Here there are *new data*. This possibility has now been tested in an RCT by WHO (2003). As shown in Table 10, the failure rate was low: only eight failures in 314 women treated between 72 and 120 hours (5 days) after the earliest act of unprotected intercourse. This is a small study and the confidence intervals are wide. But unlike FGD 2003, I would say that this makes it sufficiently evidence-based (though not yet licensed, p. 141) for POEC to be offered to selected women in the 72–120 hour time period. It is 'highly likely to be better than doing nothing', yet the woman must be informed also that a copper IUD would definitely be more effective. Neither method should be used if calculations suggest that any earlier act could have led to the presence by now of an early implanted pregnancy.
- **Overdue injections of DMPA with continuing sexual intercourse** (see p. 84). If it is later than day 91 (end of the 13th week) after a negative sensitive pregnancy test, along with the injection we give EC by hormone or more rarely a copper IUD as appropriate *plus* advice to use condoms for 7 days. But after day 98 (14 weeks), the next injection is best postponed until there has been a total of 14 days of safe contraception or

abstinence since the last exposure and a sensitive (25 mIU/l) pregnancy test is negative (see p. 46, footnote).

- **Advanced provision of POEC**; to quote FGD 2003 again, with instructions on use and how to access services if side effects should occur, this can be appropriately offered to those attending primary care or sexual and reproductive health services.

In all circumstances of use of EC, always counsel the women regarding possible failure and provide no guarantee that any fetus will be normal. Research continues and alternatives may supersede the current methods in due course.

Other reversible methods*

Barrier methods

Barrier methods are not yet out of fashion! In spite of well-known disadvantages they all (notably condoms) provide useful protection against STIs. *All users of this type of method should be informed about EC, in case of lack of use or failure in use.*

Vegetable- and oil-based lubricants, and the bases for many prescribable vaginal products, can seriously damage and lead to rupture of rubber: baby oil destroys up to 95% of a condom's strength within 15 minutes. Beware *ad hoc* use of, or contamination by substances from the kitchen or bathroom cupboard! Water-based products such as KY jelly, and also glycerine and silicone lubricants, are not suspect. The Box on page 133 lists some common vaginal preparations which should be regarded as unsafe to use with rubber condoms and diaphragms, and there may be others.

*Male and female sterilization, especially the former, are useful options for some couples: but not in the remit of this particular book

Preparations unsafe to use with rubber condoms or diaphragms	
Arachis oil enema	Gyno-Pevaryl™ (Janssen-Cilag)
Baby oil	Lomexin (Akita)
Canesten (Bayer)	Nizoral™ (Janssen Cilag)
Cyclogest™	Nystan cream™ (Bristol-Meyers
(Shire Pharmaceuticals)	Squibb) (pessaries okay)
Dalacin cream™	Ortho-Gynest™ (Janssen-Cilag)
(Pharmacia & Upjohn)	(Organon laboratories)
E45 and similar emollients	Petroleum Jelly
Ecostatin™	Sultrin (Janssen-Cilag)
(Bristol-Meyers Squibb)	Vaseline™ (Elida Faborgé)
Gyno-Daktarin™ (Janssen-Cilag)	Witepsol-based preparations

This problem does not affect plastic condoms such as Avanti and Ez-On (see below). However, there is no evidence that either of these is any less likely to rupture for mechanical reasons.

Condoms

Condoms are the only proven barrier to transmission of HIV, yet at the time of writing it still remains impossible in the UK for most couples to obtain this life-saver free of charge from every GP. Condoms are second in usage to the Pill under the age of 30 and to sterilization above that age. One GP has reported a failure rate as low as 0.4 per 100 woman-years, but 2–15 is more representative. Failure, often unrecognized at the time, can almost always be attributed to incorrect use, mainly through escape of a small amount of semen either before or after the main ejaculation. Conceptions, particularly among the young or those who have become a bit casual after years of using a simple method such as the COC, can sometimes be iatrogenic because of lack of explanation by a nurse or doctor of the basics.

Some users are entirely satisfied with the condom, whereas others use it as a temporary or back-up method. For many who have become accustomed to alternatives not related to intercourse it is completely unacceptable.

Some older men, or those with sexual anxiety, complain that its use may result in loss of erection. I consider this sometimes gives adequate grounds to prescribe sildenafil. For women who dislike the smell or messiness of semen, the condom solves their problem.

True rubber allergy can also occur (rarely) but is often solved by switching to plastic condoms (e.g. Avanti or Ez-On). If the allergy proves to be to the lubricant, if it contains nonoxynol-9 it should not be being used in the first place. Lubricants with this spermicide should be avoided with any condom, since it is now evidence-based that it can increase HIV transmission (see below) – and anyway, it provides no detectable increase in condom efficacy.

The new Ez-On condom recently marketed in the UK (by mail order from: FP Sales Ltd 01865 719400 or visit www.fpsales.co.uk) is a loose-fitting well-lubricated plastic condom – the 'looks funny, feels good' condom. By better simulating the vagina it is designed to overcome the undeniable interference with penile sensation that occurs during the penetration phase of intercourse.

Femidom

Femidom (Figure 21) is a female condom comprising a polyurethane sac with an outer rim at the introitus and a loose inner ring, whose retaining action is similar to that of the rim of the diaphragm. It thus forms a well-lubricated secondary vagina. Available over the counter, along with a well-illustrated leaflet, it is considerably less likely than most male condoms to rupture in use. It is also completely resistant to damage by any chemicals with which it might come into contact. Using it, the penetrative phase of intercourse can feel more normal (like with Ez-On) and also start before the man's erection is complete. However, couples should be forewarned of the possibility that the penis may become wrongly positioned between the Femidom sac and the vaginal wall.

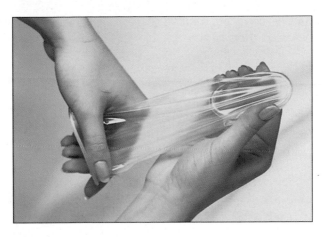

Figure 21
The female condom (Femidom). (Reproduced with kind permission of Chartex International plc.)

Reports about its acceptability are mixed, and a sense of humour certainly helps. There is evidence of a group of women (and their partners) who use it regularly; sometimes alternating with the male equivalent ('his' night then 'her' night). Others might choose it if it were more often mentioned by providers as even being an option. As the first female-controlled method with high potential for preventing HIV transmission it must be welcomed.

The cap or diaphragm
Once initiated, many couples express surprise at the simplicity of these vaginal barriers, although they are often acceptable only when sexual activity takes on a relatively regular pattern in a stable relationship. It may be inserted well ahead of coitus, and so used without spoiling spontaneity. There is very little reduction in sexual sensitivity, as the clitoris and introitus are not affected and cervical pressure is still possible.

Spermicide is recommended because no mechanical

barrier is complete, although we still lack definitive research on this point. Possible toxic effects of nonoxynol-9 – which is unfortunately the only spermicidal agent marketed in UK – to the vaginal wall have become a real concern (see below). However, the vagina is believed to be able to recover between applications when nonoxynol-9 is used in the manner, and at the kind of average coital frequency, of diaphragm-users.

The acceptability of the *diaphragm* itself depends on how it is offered. Its first-year failure rate, now estimated as 4–8 per 100 careful and consistent users, rising to 10–18 per 100 typical users, makes it very unsuitable for most young women who would not accept pregnancy. However, it suits others who are 'spacers' of their family. And it is capable of excellent protection above the age of 35 (3 per 100 woman-years, see Table 1), provided it is as well taught and correctly and consistently used as in the Oxford/FPA study.

Lea's Shield and *Femcap* are both American inventions. The latter has some efficacy data; the reported Pearl failure rate is comparable with the diaphragm, 10.5–14.5 per 100 woman-years. It is a plastic cervical cap with a brim filling the fornices, in three sizes, intended to be provided through mainstream clinics (Supplier: Family Planning Sales, Oxford) as an alternative to the diaphragm or cervical caps. It must be used with a spermicide but is reusable, needing to be replaced about every 2 years.

When there is great difficulty in inserting anything into the vagina, be it tampon, pessaries or a cap, obviously the method is not suitable. This problem may be connected with a psychosexual difficulty which may first present during the teaching of the method, but simple lack of anatomical knowledge is often involved. Rejection of a vaginal barrier on account of 'messiness' may also be the result of such a problem. The offer of a less wet-feeling alternative for the spermicide may then help, especially Delfen foam.

Follow-up

Vaginal barriers should be checked initially after 1–2 weeks of trial, then annually. The fitting of diaphragms should be re-checked routinely postpartum, or if there is a 4 kg gain or loss in weight.

If either partner returns complaining that they can feel any kind of cap during coitus the fitting must be urgently checked. It could be too large or too small; or with the diaphragm the retropubic ledge may be insufficient to prevent the front slipping down the anterior vagina; or, most seriously, the item may be being placed regularly in the anterior fornix. The *arcing spring diaphragm* is then particularly useful.

Chronic cystitis may be exacerbated by pressure from a diaphragm's anterior rim, and the condition was shown to occur less frequently with *Femcap* in the comparative pre-marketing trials. Similarly, it often improves with a *vault* or *cervical cap.*

As for the IUD, for those nurses or doctors who wish to offer this choice there is no substitute for one-to-one training, both in the process of fitting the diaphragm and cervical caps, and in teaching a woman how to use it correctly, backed by an appropriate leaflet.

With each of these products, the old type or the new, like Femcap, the single most important thing the woman must learn is the vital regular secondary check, after placing it, that she has covered her cervix correctly. Female barriers can be used happily and very successfully by many couples, but high motivation is essential. Once again, a good sense of humour helps.

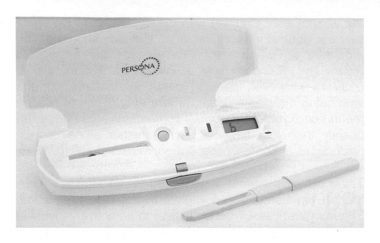

Figure 22
Persona (by courtesy of Unipath Ltd).

- to use condoms on the pre-ovulatory 'green days', this being what I call the 'amber' phase (always less 'safe' because of the capriciousness of sperm survival in a woman);
- to abstain on all 'red days';
- to have unprotected intercourse only in the post-ovulatory green phase.

If the method is to be used after *any pregnancy* or *any hormone treatment* – even just one course of hormonal EC – another method must first be used until there have been two normal cycles of an acceptable length (23–35 days).

See also p. 75 for the LAM, another 'natural' option for some to consider, through to up to 6 months postpartum.

Much more, including details of locally available *natural family planning* teachers, can be obtained from the excellent website www.fertilityuk.org.

Appendix

Use of licensed products in an unlicensed way

Whenever licensing procedures have not yet caught up with what is widely considered the best evidence-based practice, such use is quite often necessary for optimal contraceptive care, and is legitimate, provided certain criteria are observed. These are well established [See Mann R. (1991) In: (Goldberg A, Dodds-Smith I, eds) *Pharmaceutical Medicine and the Law*. RCP: London, 103–10].

The prescribing physician must:

- Adopt a practice endorsed by a responsible body of professional opinion
- Ensure good practice, including follow-up, to comply with professional indemnity requirements. *Note: this will often mean the doctor providing dedicated written materials, because the manufacturer's insert does not apply*
- **Explain to the individual that it is an unlicensed prescription**
- Give a clear account of the risks and the benefits
- **Obtain informed (verbal) consent and record this and the discussion in full**
- **Keep a separate record of the patient's details**

This is generally termed named-patient prescribing.
NB: attention to detail is exceptionally important, as in the (unlikely) event of a claim the manufacturer can be excused from any liability.

Some common examples of named-patient prescribing
- Advising more than the usual dosage: when enzyme-inducers are being used with COC (p. 63) or POP (p. 75) or hormonal EC (p. 70).
- Use of add-back oestrogen along with DMPA (p. 86), in rare and highly selected cases to treat diagnosed hypo-oestrogenism
- Use of *banded* copper IUDs for longer than licensed under the age of 40 (T-Safe Cu 380A for more than 8 years, GyneFix for more than 5 years), and above the age of 40 any copper device used until the menopause. (p. 109).
- Use of the LNG IUS above the age of 40 for more than 5 years for contraception (**not** with HRT however), at a patient's fully informed request (p. 114)
- Use of the LNG IUS as part of HRT (p. 113)
- Use of hormonal EC beyond 72 hours after the earliest exposure or more than once in a cycle (p. 130)
- Use of 'Quick start' commencement of pills or other medical methods of contraception late in the menstrual cycle, including after hormonal EC (pp. 46, 73, 128)

There are certainly others which you may identify elsewhere in this book or in your own contraceptive practice

Equivalent proprietary names for combined pills worldwide

In the previous editions of this book the above directory appeared in printed form. It listed details of the equivalent brand names used worldwide, identical with or very similar to currently marketed UK low-dose combined pills. It was based, with permission, on the *Directory of Hormonal Contraceptives*, 3rd edn [Kleinman R (ed) (1996) International Planned Parenthood Federation (IPPF)]. However, the IPPF has now put this directory in its entirety on its website. This is accessible to all (no password), accurate, and regularly updated. As it is so easy to access, the decision has been made not to produce a printed version in this edition, instead visit: www.ippf.org.uk.

Believable websites in reproductive health

www.margaretpyke.org
Training Courses on offer plus useful search engine for the most common frequently asked questions (FAQs)

www.ippf.org.uk
Online version of the Directory of Hormonal Contraception with names of (equivalent) pill brands used throughout the world

www.who.int/reproductive-health
WHO's Eligibility Criteria and new Practice Recommendations

www.rcog.org.uk
Evidence-based Royal College guidelines on male and female sterilization, infertility and menorrhagia

www.ffprhc.org.uk
Includes Faculty Guidance on Emergency Contraception, FACT reports, access to the *Journal of the Faculty of Family Planning and Reproductive Health Care*

www.fpa.org.uk
Patient information plus those essential leaflets! Also invaluable Helpline 0845 310 1334

www.fertilityuk.org
The fertility awareness and NFP service, including teachers available locally

www.agum.org.uk
National guidelines for the management of all STIs and a listing of all GUM Clinics in the UK; through a merger, AGUM has now (2003) become BASHH, the British Association for Sexual Health and HIV.

www.ruthinking.co.uk
Sex – are you thinking about it enough? Website that fully informs plus makes it really easy for teens to access services. Supported by the Teenage Pregnancy Unit

www.likeitis.org.uk
Reproductive health for lay persons by Marie Stopes and fronted by Geri Halliwell

www.teenagehealthfreak.com
FAQs as asked by teenagers, on all health subjects, not just reproductive health – from anorexia to zits!

www.the-bms.org
Research-based advice about the menopause and hormone replacement therapy (HRT).

www.ipm.org.uk
Website of the Institute of Psychosexual Medicine

www.basrt.org.uk
Website of the British Association for Sexual and Relationship Therapy; provides a list of therapists.

www.relate.org.uk
Enter postcode to get nearest Relate centre for relationship counselling and psychosexual therapy. Many publications also available.

www.ecotimecapsule.com
www.optimumpopulation.org
www.peopleandplanet.net
www. elephantintheroom.com
} John Guillebaud's website re: the *Apology to Future* project – and related sites.

Further reading

Filshie M, Guillebaud J (1989) *Contraception: Science and Practice*. Butterworths: London.

Guillebaud J (2004) *Contraception – Your Questions Answered*. Churchill-Livingstone: Edinburgh.

Guillebaud J (2003) *Contraception* In: (McPherson A, Waller D, eds) *Women's Health*, 5th edn. Oxford University Press: Oxford. [Formerly *Women's Problems in General Practice*.]

Kubba A, Sanfilippo J, Hampton N (1999) *Contraception and Office Gynaecology: Choices in Reproductive Healthcare*. WB Saunders: London.

Potts M, Diggory P (1983) *Textbook of Contraceptive Practice*. Cambridge University Press: Cambridge.

Sapire E (1990) *Contraception and Sexuality in Health and Disease*. McGraw-Hill: Isando.

WHO (2000) *Medical Eligibility Criteria for Contraceptive Use* (WHO/RHR/00.02). WHO, Geneva.

WHO (2002) *Selected Practice Recommendations for Contraceptive Use*. (ISBN: 92 4 154566 6). WHO: Geneva.

Background reading

This includes titles for a general readership.

Cooper A, Guillebaud J (1999) *Sexuality and Disability.* Radcliffe Medical Press: London.

Djerassi C (1981) *The Politics of Contraception: Birth Control in the Year 2001*, 2nd edn. Freeman: Oxford.

Ehrlich P, Ehrlich A (1991) *The Population Explosion.* Arrow Books: London.

Guillebaud J (2004) *The Pill*, 6th edn. Oxford University Press: Oxford.

Montford H, Skrine R (1993) *Psychosexual Medicine Series 6. Contraceptive Care: Meeting Individual Needs.* Chapman & Hall: London.

Population Reports (various years to 2003) Excellent comprehensive reviews of the literature on developments in population, contraception and sterilisation. www.jhuccp.org.

Skrine R, Montford H (2001) *Psychosexual medicine – an introduction.* Arnold: London.

Szarewski A, Guillebaud J (2000) *Contraception – A User's Handbook*, 3rd edn. Oxford University Press: Oxford.

Many more relevant book titles, videos and useful patient leaflets concerning all methods can be obtained by easy mail order. Contact: FPA Direct, Unit 9, Ledgers Close, Littlemore, Oxford OX4 5JS (tel 01865 719418; fax 01865 748746). Leaflets and instructions in languages other than English are also obtainable from the FPA and the International Planned Parenthood Federation, Regent's College, Inner Circle, Regent's Park, London NW1 4NS, and also through some manufacturers.

Glossary

ALO	*Actinomyces*-like organisms
AMI	acute myocardial infarction
BBD	benign breast disease
BMI	body mass index
BNF	British National Formulary
BP	blood pressure
BTB	breakthrough bleeding
CGHFBC	Collaborative Group on Hormonal Factors in Breast Cancer
CIN	cervical intraepithelial neoplasia
COC	combined oral contraception/ive
COEC	combined oral emergency contraceptive
CPA	cyproterone acetate
CSM	Committee on the Safety of Medicines [UK]
CVS	cardiovascular system
DFFP	Diploma of the Faculty of FP
DM	diabetes mellitus

DMPA	Depot medroxyprogesterone acetate (Depo-Provera)
DNA	deoxyribonucleic acid
DoH	Department of Health (now termed DH)
DSG	desogestrel
DSP	drospirenone
EC	emergency contraception
EE	ethinylestradiol
EVA	ethylene vinyl acetate
Faculty of FP	Faculty of Family Planning and Reproductive Health Care
FAQ	frequently asked question
FGD 2003	Faculty Guidance Document 2003
FPA	Family Planning Association
FSH	follicle-stimulating hormone
GP	general practitioner
GSD	gestodene
GUM	genitourinary medicine
hCG	human chorionic gonadotrophin
HDL	high-density lipoprotein
HIV	human immunodeficiency virus
HPV	human papilloma virus
HRT	hormone replacement therapy
HUS	haemolytic uraemic syndrome
INR	International normalized ratio – blood test used to control warfarin anticoagulant level
IPPF	International Planned Parenthood Federation
IUD	intrauterine device
IUS	intrauterine system
LAM	lactational amenorrhoea method
LCR	ligase chain reaction – ultrasensitive & specific test (e.g. for Chlamydia)
LMP	last menstrual period
LNG IUS	levonorgestrel IUS
MFFP	Membership of the Faculty of FP
MPC	Margaret Pyke Centre
NET	norethisterone (termed norethindrone in the US)
NETA	norethisterone acetate
NGM	norgestimate
PCOS	polycystic ovarian syndrome
PCR	polymerase chain reaction (like LCR, for ultrasensitive/specific tests)
PFI	pill-free interval
PID	pelvic inflammatory disease
PMS	premenstrual syndrome
POEC	progestogen-only emergency contraceptive
POP	progestogen-only pill
RCGP	Royal College of GPs
RCN	Royal College of Nursing
RCOG	Royal College of Obstetricians & Gynaecologists
RCT	randomized controlled trial

SHGB	sex-hormone binding globulin
SLE	systemic lupus erythematosus
SPC	Summary of Product Characteristics (= Data Sheet)
SRE	sex and relationships education
STI	sexually transmitted infection
TTP	thrombotic thrombocytopenic purpura
UPSI	unprotected sexual intercourse
VTE	venous thromboembolism
WHO	World Health Organization

Coventry University

Index